W9-BZS-113

CONCISE GUIDE TO

Psychopharmacology

Second Edition

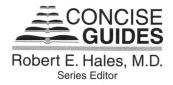

CONCISE GUIDES

Robert E. Hales, M.D.
Series Editor

CONCISE GUIDE TO
Psychopharmacology

Second Edition

Lauren B. Marangell, M.D.

James M. Martinez, M.D.

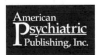

American **P**sychiatric Publishing, Inc.

Washington, DC
London, England

Note: The authors have worked to ensure that all information in this book is accurate at the time of publication and consistent with general psychiatric and medical standards, and that information concerning drug dosages, schedules, and routes of administration is accurate at the time of publication and consistent with standards set by the U.S. Food and Drug Administration and the general medical community. As medical research and practice advance, however, therapeutic standards may change. Moreover, specific situations may require a specific therapeutic response not included in this book. For these reasons and because human and mechanical errors sometimes occur, we recommend that readers follow the advice of physicians directly involved in their care or the care of a member of their family. A product's current package insert should be consulted for full prescribing and safety information.

Copyright © 2006 American Psychiatric Publishing, Inc.
ALL RIGHTS RESERVED

This Concise Guide was developed in part from Marangell LB, Silver JM, Goff DC, et al: "Psychopharmacology and ECT," in *The American Psychiatric Publishing Textbook of Clinical Psychiatry,* Fourth Edition. Edited by Hales RE, Yudofsky SC. Washington, DC, American Psychiatric Publishing, 2002. Used with permission.

Manufactured in the United States of America on acid-free paper
10   09   08   07   06   5   4   3   2   1
Second Edition

American Psychiatric Publishing, Inc.
1000 Wilson Boulevard
Arlington, VA 22209-3901
www.appi.org

To purchase 25–99 copies of any APPI title at a 20% discount, please contact APPI Customer Service at appi@psych.org or 800-368-5777. To purchase 100 or more copies of the same title, please e-mail bulksales@psych.org for a price quote.

Library of Congress Cataloging-in-Publication Data
Marangell, Lauren B., 1961-
    Concise guide to psychopharmacology / Lauren B. Marangell, James M. Martinez. -- 2nd ed.
        p. ; cm. -- (Concise guides series)
    Rev. ed. of: Concise guide to psychopharmacology / Lauren B. Marangell ... [et al.]. 1st ed. c2002.
    Includes bibliographical references and index.
    ISBN 1-58562-255-9 (pbk. : alk. paper)
    1. Psychopharmacology--Handbooks, manuals, etc. I. Martinez, James M. II. American Psychiatric Publishing. III. Concise guide to psychopharmacology. IV. Title. V. Title: Psychopharmacology.
    VI. Series: Concise guides (American Psychiatric Publishing)
    [DNLM: 1. Psychotropic Drugs--therapeutic use--Practice Guideline. 2. Mental Disorders--drug therapy--Practice Guideline. 3. Psycho-pharmacology--methods--Practice Guideline.
    QV 77.2 M311c 2006]
    RM315.C596 2006
    615'.78--dc22

                                                                                          2005035237

British Library Cataloguing in Publication Data
A CIP record is available from the British Library.

CONTENTS

3 Anxiolytics, Sedatives, and Hypnotics 69

LIST OF TABLES

ABOUT THE AUTHORS

Lauren B. Marangell, M.D., is the Brown Foundation Chair of the Psychopharmacology of Mood Disorders, Associate Professor of Psychiatry, and Director of Mood Disorders Research in the Menninger Department of Psychiatry at Baylor College of Medicine in Houston, Texas.

James M. Martinez, M.D., is Associate Director of the Mood Disorders Program and Assistant Professor of Psychiatry in the Menninger Department of Psychiatry at Baylor College of Medicine in Houston, Texas.

INTRODUCTION

to the Concise Guides Series

The Concise Guides Series from American Psychiatric Publishing, Inc., provides, in an accessible format, practical information for psychiatrists, psychiatry residents, and medical students working in a variety of treatment settings, such as inpatient psychiatry units, outpatient clinics, consultation-liaison services, and private offices. The Concise Guides are meant to complement the more detailed information to be found in lengthier psychiatry texts.

The Concise Guides address topics of special concern to psychiatrists in clinical practice. The books in this series contain a detailed table of contents, along with an index, tables, figures, and other charts for easy access. The books are designed to fit into a laboratory coat pocket or jacket pocket, which makes them a convenient source of information. References have been limited to those most relevant to the material presented.

Robert E. Hales, M.D., M.B.A.
Series Editor, American Psychiatric Publishing Concise Guides

ACKNOWLEDGMENTS

This book is dedicated to our children, Jonathan, Elizabeth, Cameron, and Connor. We especially acknowledge Stuart C. Yudofsky, M.D., and Jonathan M. Silver, M.D., who were coauthors of the first edition of the *Concise Guide to Psychopharmacology* and the chapter on psychopharmacology in the *American Psychiatric Publishing Textbook of Psychiatry,* in which this work had its genesis.

GENERAL PRINCIPLES

Skillful practice of psychopharmacology requires a broad knowledge of psychiatry, pharmacology, and medicine. In this chapter, we present general principles relevant to the safe and effective use of psychotropic medications. In subsequent chapters, we discuss the major classes of psychotropic medications—antidepressants, anxiolytics, antipsychotics, mood stabilizers, stimulants, and cognitive enhancers—and the disorders for which they are prescribed. The reader should be aware that this nomenclature is somewhat artificial; for example, many antidepressant medications are also used to treat anxiety disorders. Generic names are used throughout this book. The appendix provides a list of trade (brand) names.

■ INITIAL EVALUATION

The art of psychopharmacology, like that of all areas of medicine, rests on proper diagnosis and delineation of medication-responsive target symptoms. Additional aspects include ruling out nonpsychiatric causes, such as endocrine or neurological disorders and substance abuse; noting the presence of other medical problems that will influence drug selection, such as cardiac or hepatic disease; evaluating other medications that the patient is taking that might cause a drug-drug interaction; and evaluating personal and family histories of medication responses.

■ TARGET SYMPTOMS

A key component of a well-considered decision to use a medication is the delineation of target symptoms. The physician should determine and list the specific symptoms that are designated for treatment, and he or she should monitor the response of these symptoms to treatment. Standard rating scales are specific tools for assessing symptoms and target behaviors and are useful for monitoring change with treatment. In the absence of formal rating scales, target symptoms can be rated on a 1–10 scale. In addition, the clinician should monitor functional status. The goal of treatment is not only to alleviate symptoms but also to restore normal functioning to the extent possible.

■ USE OF MULTIPLE MEDICATIONS

A frequent and dangerous clinical error is to treat specific symptoms of a disorder with multiple drugs rather than to treat the underlying disorder itself. For example, it is not uncommon for a psychiatrist to see a referred patient who is taking one type of benzodiazepine for anxiety, a different type of benzodiazepine for insomnia, an analgesic for nonspecific somatic complaints, and a subtherapeutic dose of an antidepressant (e.g., imipramine 50 mg/day) for feelings of sadness. Often, the somatic complaints, insomnia, and anxiety are components of an underlying depression, which may be aggravated by the polypharmaceutical approach inherent in symptomatic treatment.

Conversely, many patients have psychiatric conditions that require the concomitant use of several psychotropic agents. The carefully considered, rational use of several psychiatric medications must be distinguished from ill-considered polypharmacy. An example of useful combined treatment is the addition of lithium to antidepressant therapy in the case of a patient who has achieved only a partial response to treatment with an antidepressant alone.

■ CHOICE OF DRUG

Selection of a drug for a given diagnosis or symptom is based on both patient-specific and drug-specific factors. Patient-specific factors include comorbid medical and psychiatric disorders, other medications being taken, history of response to medication, family history of medication response, and life circumstances that likely will be affected by the side effects of the chosen agent. Drug-specific factors include available preparations and cost. In most cases, once-daily dosing is preferred, for patient convenience and treatment adherence.

■ GENERIC SUBSTITUTION

Generic drugs are less expensive alternatives to original proprietary (brand name) formulations. However, some caution is warranted because generic "equivalents" are not always truly equivalent. Therefore, increased clinical scrutiny of both exacerbation of psychiatric symptoms and new side effects is warranted when changing from a brand-name product to a generic preparation. The current U.S. Food and Drug Administration requirements center on the concept of *bioequivalence*. Products are bioequivalent if there is no significant difference in the rate at which or extent to which the active ingredient becomes available at the site of action, given the same dose and conditions. In some cases, however, even small differences in bioavailability—or other small differences, such as in the type of preservatives or excipients—may become clinically meaningful. For example, a patient may have an allergic reaction to one generic preparation but not another of the same drug because of differences in the dye used to color the pill.

In many circumstances, generic substitution is a safe and effective cost-saving tool, but the clinician should be aware of potential problems and, in the event of an unexpected reaction, should ask the patient if the medication has changed in appearance. A change in size, shape, or color, for example, should alert the clinician to a probable change in generic formulation.

■ DRUG INTERACTIONS

A drug interaction occurs when the pharmacological action of a medication is altered by a concurrently administered drug (or exogenous substance). With the increased use of psychotropic medications, the importance of drug interactions in psychopharmacology is increasingly apparent. Also, the characterization of specific cytochrome P450 (CYP) enzymes has made it possible to understand and predict many drug-drug interactions.

There are three types of drug interactions. *Pharmacokinetic interactions* involve an alteration by a second agent in the absorption, distribution, metabolism, or excretion of a drug, which changes the plasma concentration of the drug. *Pharmacodynamic interactions* involve a change in the action of a drug at a receptor or biologically active site, which alters the pharmacological effect of a given plasma concentration of the drug. *Idiosyncratic interactions* occur unpredictably in a few patients; they are unexpected, given the known pharmacological actions of the individual drugs.

Cytochrome P450 Enzymes

Clinically significant drug interactions are most commonly caused by changes in drug metabolism. Cytochrome P450 enzymes metabolize most psychotropic drugs except lithium. These enzymes are classified by families and subfamilies on the basis of similarities in amino acid sequence. Enzymes within subfamilies have relatively specific affinities for various drugs and other substances. The enzymes primarily involved in drug metabolism are CYP 1A2, 2C9, 2C10, 2C19, 2D6, 3A3, and 3A4.

If one of these enzymes is inhibited by another drug, then the plasma levels of the concurrently administered drugs that rely on the enzyme for metabolism increase. For example, 2D6 is essential for the usual metabolism of tricyclic antidepressants (TCAs), which are substrates for this enzyme. Paroxetine inhibits 2D6. If a patient is taking a TCA and paroxetine is added, or vice versa, plasma TCA levels increase, which may result in increased TCA-related side effects or toxicity. Aware of the potential for this reaction, the clinician might use a lower dose of the TCA. This example illustrates the key clinical principle of prescribing enzyme inhibitors: in most cases, the combination of an enzyme inhibitor and a medication that is a substrate for that enzyme is not contraindicated, but the patient should be monitored for signs and symptoms related to increased substrate levels, and the substrate dose should be decreased if necessary. With regard to many medications, the specific cytochrome P450 enzymes responsible for metabolism are not yet known, but information about the role of cytochrome P450 enzymes in drug metabolism is rapidly accumulating. Table 1–1 is a list of the better-recognized and clinically important substrates for and inhibitors of the cytochrome P450 enzymes most commonly involved in drug metabolism. In most cases, enzyme inhibitors and substrates can be safely combined, provided the dose of the substrate is decreased as needed.

The effects of inhibitors occur relatively rapidly (in minutes to hours) and are reversible within a time frame that depends on the half-life of the inhibitor. There is a large amount of interindividual variation in drug metabolism and the propensity for enzyme inhibition to alter metabolism. Part of this variation is the result of genetic polymorphism, which is a heritable alteration of the enzyme. Cytochrome P450 enzymes 2C19 and 2D6 are known to show polymorphism. Persons who have a genetic polymorphism that causes a large reduction in the amount of active enzyme are referred to as *poor metabolizers* and are at risk for increased drug levels, which may lead to toxicity. In contrast, some people have increased amounts of an enzyme. These individuals, referred to as *ultrarapid metabolizers,* may have reduced levels of drugs that are metabolized by the enzyme, resulting in decreased efficacy. Polymorphism accounts for many of the well-known interindividual differences in drug metabolism and the drug-drug interactions mediated by cytochrome P450 enzymes.

In addition, many of the cytochrome P450 enzymes can be induced. Induction causes the liver to produce a greater amount of the enzyme, which can increase elimination and reduce plasma levels

TABLE 1–1. Partial list of clinically relevant cytochrome P450 substrates and inhibitors

	CYP 1A2	CYP 2D6	CYP 3A4
Substrates[a]	Aminophylline	Most antipsychotics	Acetaminophen
	Amitriptyline	Amphetamine	Alprazolam
	Caffeine	Codeine	Amiodarone
	Clozapine (in part)	Donepezil	Antiarrhythmics
	Cyclobenzaprine	Encainide	Calcium channel blockers
	Flutamide	Flecainide	Carbamazepine
	Imipramine	Galantamine	Cyclosporine
	Riluzole	Lipophilic β-blockers	Donepezil
	Ramelteon	Mexiletine	Eszopiclone
	Theophylline	Oxycodone	Ethosuximide
		Tricyclic antidepressants[b]	Galantamine
		Tramadol	HMG-CoA reductase inhibitors (e.g., atorvastatin)
		Trazodone	Lamotrigine
		Type IC antiarrhythmics	Lidocaine
		Venlafaxine	Midazolam
			Most antineoplastics
			Oral contraceptives
			Oxcarbazepine
			Phosphodiesterase inhibitors (e.g., sildenafil)

TABLE 1–1. Partial list of clinically relevant cytochrome P450 substrates and inhibitors *(continued)*

	CYP 1A2	CYP 2D6	CYP 3A3/4
Substrates *(continued)*			Pimozide
			Propafenone
			Protease inhibitors (e.g., ritonavir)
			Quinidine
			Steroids
			Zaleplon
			Zolpidem
			CYP 3A3/4/5
			Diltiazem
			Fluvoxamine
			Grapefruit juice
			Imidazole antifungal agents (e.g., ketoconazole)
			Some macrolides (e.g., azithromycin)
			Nefazodone
			Protease inhibitors
			Verapamil
Inhibitors[c]	Cimetidine	Bupropion	
	Ciprofloxacin	Cimetidine	
	Enoxacin	Diloxetine	
	Flutamide	Fluoxetine	
	Fluvoxamine	Paroxetine	
	Grapefruit juice	Quinidine	
	Ketoconazole	Ritonavir	
	Lomefloxacin	Sertraline	
	Norfloxacin		

Note. CYP=cytochrome P450; HMG-CoA=3-hydroxy-3-methylglutaryl coenzyme A.
[a] Medications and substances metabolized by a given enzyme.
[b] The 2D6 enzyme is the final common pathway for the metabolism of tricyclic antidepressants.
[c] May increase levels of substrates.
Source. Callahan et al. 1996; Cozza et al. 2003; Greenblatt et al. 1998, 1999; Michalets 1998.

of a second drug or its metabolites. If a reduction in a drug's plasma level diminishes its clinical effectiveness, then the dose of the affected drug should be increased to achieve the same serum concentration. The effects of inducers tend to be delayed for days to weeks because this process involves enzyme synthesis. Barbiturates, carbamazepine, phenytoin, rifampin, dexamethasone, smoking, and chronic alcohol use induce cytochrome P450 enzymes. St. John's wort has been reported to decrease levels and/or the effectiveness of cyclosporine (Ahmed et al. 2001; Breidenbach et al. 2000; Karliova et al. 2000) and protease inhibitors (Durr et al. 2000). Some enzyme-inducing medications often used in the treatment of psychiatric disorders include carbamazepine, oxcarbazepine, and modafinil. Additionally, topiramate may decrease the efficacy of oral contraceptives containing ethinyl estradiol (Cozza et al. 2003).

Protein Binding

Medications are distributed to their sites of action through the circulatory system. In the bloodstream, all psychotropic medications except lithium are bound to plasma proteins to varying degrees. A drug is considered highly protein bound if more than 90% of the drug is bound to plasma proteins. A reversible equilibrium exists between the bound and unbound drug: the unbound fraction is pharmacologically active, whereas the bound fraction is inactive and therefore cannot be metabolized or excreted. When two drugs exist simultaneously in the plasma, competition for protein binding sites occurs. This can cause displacement of the previously protein-bound drug, which in the free state becomes pharmacologically active. Interactions that occur by this mechanism are called *protein-binding interactions*. They are transient; although the plasma concentration of free drug initially increases, the drug becomes subject to redistribution, metabolism, and excretion, producing a new steady-state concentration. This type of interaction is generally not clinically significant unless the drugs involved are highly protein bound (which results in a large change in plasma concentration of free drug from a small amount of drug displacement) and have a low therapeutic index or narrow therapeutic window (in which case small changes in plasma levels can result in toxicity or loss of efficacy) (Callahan et al. 1996).

Absorption and Excretion

Changes in plasma levels as a result of alterations in absorption or excretion are less common with psychiatric medications. Changes in plasma concentrations as a result of changes in excretion are most frequent with lithium, which is dependent on renal excretion (see Chapter 5).

Pharmacodynamic Interactions

In pharmacodynamic interactions, the pharmacological effect of a drug is changed by the action of a second drug at a common receptor or bioactive site. For example, low-potency antipsychotics and tertiary amine TCAs have anticholinergic, antihistaminic, α-adrenergic antagonist, and quinidine-like effects. Therefore, concurrent administration of chlorpromazine and imipramine results in additive sedation, constipation, postural hypotension, and depression of cardiac conduction.

■ REFERENCES

Ahmed SM, Banner NR, Dubrey SW: Low cyclosporin-A level due to Saint-John's-wort in heart transplant patients (letter). J Heart Lung Transplant 20:795, 2001

Breidenbach T, Hoffmann MW, Becker T, et al: Drug interaction of St John's wort with cyclosporin (letter). Lancet 355:1912, 2000

Callahan AM, Marangell LB, Ketter TA: Evaluating the clinical significance of drug interactions: a systematic approach. Harv Rev Psychiatry 4:153–158, 1996

Cozza KL, Armstrong SC, Oesterheld JR: Concise Guide to Drug Interaction Principles for Medical Practice: Cytochrome P450s, UGTs, P-Glycoproteins, 2nd Edition. Washington, DC, American Psychiatric Publishing, 2003

Durr D, Stieger B, Kullak-Ublick GA, et al: St John's wort induces intestinal P-glycoprotein/MDR1 and intestinal and hepatic CYP3A4. Clin Pharmacol Ther 68:598–604, 2000

Greenblatt DJ, von Moltke LL, Harmatz JS, et al: Drug interactions with newer antidepressants: role of human cytochromes P450. J Clin Psychiatry 59 (suppl 15):19–27, 1998

Greenblatt DJ, von Moltke LL, Harmatz JS, et al: Human cytochromes and some newer antidepressants: kinetics, metabolism, and drug interactions. J Clin Psychopharmacol 19:23S–35S, 1999

Karliova M, Treichel U, Malago M, et al: Interaction of *Hypericum perforatum* (St. John's wort) with cyclosporin A metabolism in a patient after liver transplantation. J Hepatol 33:853–855, 2000

Michalets EL: Update: clinically significant cytochrome P-450 drug interactions. Pharmacotherapy 18:84–112, 1998

2

ANTIDEPRESSANTS

To date, all antidepressants appear to be similarly effective for treating major depression, but individual patients may respond preferentially to one agent or another. In addition, these medications are significantly different from one another with regard to side effects, lethality in overdose, pharmacokinetics, and the ability to treat comorbid disorders.

■ MECHANISMS OF ACTION

All current antidepressant drugs affect the serotonergic and/or noradrenergic systems in the brain. The effects of antidepressants on monoamine availability are immediate, but the clinical response is typically delayed for several weeks. Downregulation of receptors more closely parallels the time course of clinical response. This downregulation can be conceptualized as a marker of antidepressant-induced neuronal adaptation. Therapeutic effects are most likely related to modulation of G proteins, second-messenger systems, and gene expression, particularly genes involved in neuronal growth and regeneration (for review, see Nestler et al. 2002).

■ INDICATIONS AND EFFICACY

Although antidepressants have many potential therapeutic uses, their primary approved indication is the treatment of major depression. Overall, approximately 65% of patients with depression respond to an adequate trial of antidepressant medication, although far fewer achieve full remission of symptoms. In addition, antidepressants are effective in patients with obsessive-compulsive disorder (OCD; selective serotonin reuptake inhibitors [SSRIs] and clomipramine), panic disorder (tricyclic antidepressants [TCAs] and SSRIs), generalized anxiety disorder (venlafaxine and SSRIs), bulimia (TCAs, SSRIs, and monoamine oxidase inhibitors [MAOIs]), dysthymia (SSRIs), bipolar depression (with treatment with a mood stabilizer), social phobia (SSRIs, venlafaxine, MAOIs), posttraumatic stress disorder (SSRIs), irritable bowel syndrome (TCAs), enuresis (TCAs), neuropathic pain (TCAs, duloxetine), migraine headaches (TCAs), attention-deficit/hyperactivity disorder (bupropion), autism (SSRIs), late luteal phase dysphoric disorder (SSRIs), or borderline personality disorder (SSRIs), as well as in smoking cessation (bupropion); however, the U.S. Food and Drug Administration has not evaluated or approved the use of antidepressants to treat many of these conditions.

■ CLINICAL USE

The commonly used classes of antidepressants are discussed in the following sections, and information about doses and half-lives is summarized in Table 2–1. The antidepressant classes are based on similarity of receptor effects and side effects. All are effective against depression when administered in therapeutic doses. The choice of antidepressant medication is based on the patient's psychiatric symptoms, his or her history of treatment response, family members' history of response, medication side-effect profiles, and comorbid disorders (Tables 2–2 and 2–3). In general, SSRIs and the other newer antidepressants are better tolerated and safer than TCAs and MAOIs, although many patients benefit from treatment with these older drugs. In the following sections, clinically relevant information is presented for the antidepressant medication classes individually, and the pharmacological treatment of depression is also discussed. The use of antidepressants to treat anxiety disorders is addressed in Chapter 3.

TABLE 2–1. Commonly used antidepressant drugs

Drug	Trade name	Starting dose (mg)[a]	Usual daily dose (mg)	Available oral doses (mg)	Mean half-life (hours)[b]
SSRIs					
Citalopram	Celexa	20	20–40[c]	10, 20, 40, L	35
Escitalopram	Lexapro	10	10–20	5, 10, 20, L	27–32
Fluoxetine	Prozac	20	20–60[c]	10, 20, 40, L	72 (216)
Fluoxetine Weekly	Prozac Weekly	90	NA	90	—
Fluvoxamine[d]	Luvox	50	50–300[c]	25, 50, 100	15
Paroxetine	Paxil	20	20–60[c]	10, 20, 30, 40, L	20
Paroxetine CR	Paxil CR	25	25–62.5	12.5, 25, 37.5	15–20
Sertraline	Zoloft	50	50–200[c]	25, 50, 100	26 (66)
SNRIs					
Duloxetine	Cymbalta	30	60–90	20, 30, 60	12
Venlafaxine	Effexor	37.5	75–225	25, 37.5, 50, 75, 100	5 (11)
Venlafaxine XR	Effexor XR	37.5	75–225	37.5, 75, 150	5 (11)
Serotonin modulators					
Nefazodone[d]	Serzone	50	150–300	100, 150, 200, 250	4
Trazodone	Desyrel	50	75–300	50, 100, 150, 300	7

TABLE 2–1. Commonly used antidepressant drugs *(continued)*

Drug	Trade name	Starting dose (mg)[a]	Usual daily dose (mg)	Available oral doses (mg)	Mean half-life (hours)[b]
Norepinephrine-serotonin modulators					
Mirtazapine	Remeron	15	15–45	7.5, 15, 30, 45, soltab	20
Others					
Bupropion	Wellbutrin	150	300	75, 100	14
Bupropion SR	Wellbutrin SR	150	300	100, 150	21
Bupropion XL	Wellbutrin XL	300	300	100, 150	21
Tricyclics					
Tertiary amine tricyclics					
Amitriptyline	Elavil	25–50		25, 50, 75	16 (27)
Clomipramine	Anafranil	25	100–250	25, 50, 75, 100, 150, L	32 (69)
Doxepin	Sinequan	25–50	100–300	10, 25, 50, 75, 100, 150, L	17
Imipramine	Tofranil	25–50	100–300	10, 25, 50, 75, 100, 125, 150	8 (17)
Trimipramine	Surmontil	25–50	100–300	25, 50, 100	24
Secondary amine tricyclics					
Desipramine	Norpramin	25–50	100–300	10, 25, 50, 75, 100, 150	17

TABLE 2-1. Commonly used antidepressant drugs *(continued)*

Drug	Trade name	Starting dose (mg)[a]	Usual daily dose (mg)	Available oral doses (mg)	Mean half-life (hours)[b]
Nortriptyline	Pamelor, Aventyl	25	50–150	10, 25, 50, 75, L	27
Protriptyline	Vivactil	10	15–60	5, 10	79
Tetracyclics					
Amoxapine	Asendin	50	100–400	25, 50, 100, 150	8
Maprotiline	Ludiomil	50	100–225	25, 50, 75	43
MAOIs					
Irreversible, nonselective MAOIs					
Isocarboxazid	Marplan	10	20–60	10	2
Phenelzine	Nardil	15	15–90	15	2
Tranylcypromine	Parnate	10	30–60	10	2
Reversible, MAO A–selective MAOIs					
Moclobemide[c]	Aurorix, Manerix	150	300–600	100, 150	2

TABLE 2–1.   Commonly used antidepressant drugs *(continued)*

Drug	Trade name	Starting dose (mg)[a]	Usual daily dose (mg)	Available oral doses (mg)	Mean half-life (hours)[b]

Note.   L=liquid; CR=controlled release; SR=sustained-release; XR=extended-release; soltab=orally disintegrating tablets; MAOI=monoamine oxidase inhibitor; MAO A=monoamine oxidase A; SSRI=selective serotonin reuptake inhibitor; SNRI=serotonin-norepinephrine reuptake inhibitor.

[a]Lower starting doses are recommended for elderly patients and patients with panic disorder, significant anxiety, or hepatic disease.
[b]Mean half-lives of active metabolites are given in parentheses.
[c]Dose varies with diagnosis. See text for specific guidelines.
[d]Generic only.
[e]Not available in the United States.

Source.   Dosing information from American Psychiatric Association 2000. half-life data from Physicians' Desk Reference 2005.

TABLE 2–2. Guidelines for choosing antidepressant medications

Unipolar depression	Choose on the basis of previous response, side effects, and comorbid medical and psychiatric disorders.
Bipolar depression[a]	Lithium, lamotrigine, olanzapine-fluoxetine combination
Depression with psychotic features	Antidepressant+antipsychotic, or ECT; avoid bupropion
Depression+OCD	SSRI, clomipramine
Depression+panic disorder	SSRI, TCA
Depression+seizures	Avoid bupropion and TCAs
Depression+Parkinson's disease	Bupropion
Depression+sexual dysfunction	Bupropion, mirtazapine
Depression with melancholic features	TCA[b]
Depression with atypical features	SSRI, MAOI[c]

Note. ECT=electroconvulsive therapy; OCD=obsessive-compulsive disorder; SSRI=selective serotonin reuptake inhibitor; TCA=tricyclic antidepressant; MAOI=monoamine oxidase inhibitor.

[a]See Chapter 5.

[b]Although some data suggest that TCAs are superior for treating melancholic depression, most clinicians choose newer agents because of improved tolerability and safety.

[c]Although MAOIs are highly effective they are not used as first-line agents because greater risk is associated with their use than with the use of newer agents.

TABLE 2–3. Key features and side effects of antidepressant medications

Medications	Proposed mechanism/ receptor effects	Dosing	Titration required	Sedation	Weight gain	Sexual dysfunction	Other key side effects
TCAs	Serotonin+NE reuptake inhibition	Once-daily	Yes	Most, yes	Yes	Yes	Anticholinergic effects,[a] orthostasis, quinidine-like effects on cardiac conduction; lethal in overdose
SSRIs	Serotonin reuptake inhibition	Once-daily	Minimal	Minimal	Rare	Yes	Initial: nausea, loose bowel movements, headache, insomnia
Bupropion SR	DA+NE reuptake inhibition	Divided if dose >200mg	Some	Rare	Rare	Rare	Initial: nausea, headache, insomnia, anxiety or agitation; seizure risk
Venlafaxine XR	Serotonin+NE >DA reuptake inhibition	Once-daily	Yes	Minimal	Rare	Yes	Similar to SSRI side effects; dose-dependent hypertension

TABLE 2–3. Key features and side effects of antidepressant medications *(continued)*

Medications	Proposed mechanism/ receptor effects	Dosing	Titration required	Sedation	Weight gain	Sexual dysfunction	Other key side effects
Duloxetine	Serotonin+NE reuptake inhibition	Once-daily	Minimal	Minimal	Rare	Some	Initial: nausea; similar to SSRI side effects
Trazodone	5-HT$_2$ antagonism+ weak serotonin reuptake inhibition	Twice-daily	Yes	Yes	Rare	Rare	Sedation, priapism, dizziness, orthostasis
Mirtazapine	α_2-Adrenergic– 5-HT$_2$ receptor antagonism	Once-daily	Minimal	Yes	Yes	Rare	Anticholinergic effects[a], may increase serum lipid levels; rare: orthostasis, hypertension, peripheral edema, agranulocytosis

TABLE 2–3. **Key features and side effects of antidepressant medications** *(continued)*

Medications	Proposed mechanism/ receptor effects	Dosing	Titration required	Sedation	Weight gain	Sexual dysfunction	Other key side effects
MAOIs	Inhibition of MAO	Two to three times a day	Yes	Rare	Yes	Yes	Orthostatic hypotension, insomnia, peripheral edema; avoid in patients with CHF; avoid phenelzine in patients with hepatic impairment; potentially life-threatening drug interactions; dietary restrictions

Note. TCAs=tricyclic antidepressants; NE=norepinephrine; SSRIs=selective serotonin reuptake inhibitors; SR=sustained-release; DA=dopamine; XR=extended-release; 5-HT$_2$=serotonin type 2 receptor; MAOIs=monoamine oxidase inhibitors; MAO=monoamine oxidase; CHF=congestive heart failure.

[a]Anticholinergic side effects include dry mouth, blurred vision, constipation, urinary retention, tachycardia, and sometimes confusion.

Patients with depression and other psychiatric disorders are at an increased risk for suicide and suicidal behavior. Although long-term pharmacological treatment is associated with a decreased suicide rate (Angst et al. 2002), the acute phases of treatment with antidepressants have been associated with increased risks of suicidal thoughts and behaviors. This is of particular concern in children and adolescents. A pooled analysis conducted by the U.S. Food and Drug Administration (2004) of 24 short-term placebo-controlled clinical trials among children and adolescents taking antidepressants found a risk of suicidal thinking or behavior in 4% of the patients who received antidepressants, compared with 2% of the patients who received placebo. Fortunately, no suicides were completed in these studies. At this time, it is not possible to determine whether any one medication or class of medications differs with regard to the risk of early treatment–emergent suicidality; thus, warnings apply to all antidepressant medications. Although data from adult placebo-controlled trials have not been evaluated in the same systematic manner, some adult patients might be at risk in the initial weeks of treatment. These warnings are not intended to prevent the use of these medicines but rather to underscore the need for thoughtful patient education and monitoring. Specifically, the patient should be educated to call the clinician immediately if he or she experiences an increase in suicidal impulses, agitation, or severe restlessness. Family education is also warranted for pediatric patients or those with cognitive impairment.

■ SELECTIVE SEROTONIN REUPTAKE INHIBITORS

SSRIs were developed in an attempt to formulate reuptake-blocking drugs that lacked the troublesome side effects of TCAs. Of the five pharmacological properties of TCAs—blockade of muscarinic receptors, blockade of histamine H_1 receptors, blockade of α_1-adrenergic receptors, norepinephrine reuptake blockade, and serotonin reuptake inhibition—only the last remains intact in SSRIs. This selectivity has several advantages, including a reduction in dangerous side effects. SSRIs are much safer in overdose than are TCAs. In addition, SSRIs are unlikely to affect the seizure threshold or cardiac conduction.

SSRIs have an unusually broad spectrum of action. They are efficacious in the treatment not only of depression but also of many other psychiatric disorders, including many anxiety disorders. This broad spectrum of efficacy is advantageous when treating patients who have more than one disorder. For example, only SSRIs and clomipramine have been shown in randomized controlled trials to be effective in patients with OCD.

All the SSRIs have similar spectrums of efficacy and similar side-effect profiles. However, they are structurally and in some instances clinically distinct. For example, allergy to one SSRI does not predict allergy to another. Similarly, response or nonresponse to one SSRI does not necessarily predict a similar reaction to another medication in the class. SSRIs also have distinct pharmacokinetic properties, the most important of which are differences in half-life (Table 2–1) and the propensity to inhibit cytochrome P450 (CYP) enzymes (Table 1–1).

Treatment with SSRIs is started at or near their therapeutic antidepressant doses. The most significant disadvantage of these medications is a high incidence of treatment-emergent sexual dysfunction (see "Sexual Dysfunction" subsection later in this section), which often persists for as long as the patient continues taking the medication.

Clinical Use

Although all patients with depression should undergo a thorough medical evaluation, no specific tests are required before SSRI therapy is initiated. The usual starting doses of SSRIs are summarized in Table 2–1. These standard doses should be decreased by 50% in patients with hepatic disease and in elderly persons. In addition, patients with panic disorder or significant anxiety symptoms are often intolerant of the initial stimulating side effects that commonly occur with SSRI use. In these cases, the initial dose should be decreased by 50% (or more), and the dose should then be increased as tolerated to the usual therapeutic dose. It is often advantageous to apply this approach to patients who generally tend to be sensitive to side effects.

Fluoxetine was the first of the newer antidepressants to be sold in generic form in the United States; generic fluoxetine became available in 2001. A weekly formulation of fluoxetine is also available (Prozac Weekly). Administration of Prozac Weekly results in increased fluctuation between peak and trough concentrations compared with once-daily dosing. Peak concentrations reached with administration of Prozac Weekly are in the range of the average concentration achieved with 20-mg, once-daily dosing. Average steady-state concentrations achieved with once-weekly dosing are approximately 50% lower than those reached with 20-mg, once-daily dosing.

In patients with depression, SSRIs have a flat dose-response curve, meaning that higher doses tend not to be more effective than standard doses, although isolated patients respond better to higher doses. Premature escalation of the SSRI dose when treating depression is most likely to add side effects without improving antidepressant efficacy. Therefore, we recommend maintaining the usual therapeutic dose for 4 weeks. If no improvement occurs after 4 weeks, a trial of a higher dose may be warranted. If a partial response is evident after 4 weeks of therapy, the dose should remain constant for an additional 2 weeks because further improvement at the initial dose may occur.

Treatment of OCD requires a longer duration, and higher doses, to assess efficacy. A therapeutic trial for OCD should last 8–12 weeks. Treatment of anxiety disorders is discussed in Chapter 3. Late luteal phase dysphoric disorder is more responsive to serotonergic agents than to noradrenergic agents. Interestingly, late luteal phase dysphoric disorder can be treated with medication administered either only during the symptomatic period before menses or on a continuous basis (Pearlstein et al. 2000; Wikander et al. 1998; Yonkers et al. 1997).

Risks, Side Effects, and Their Management

Common Side Effects

Mild nausea, loose bowel movements, anxiety, headache, insomnia, and increased sweating are frequent initial side effects of SSRIs. They are usually dose related and may be minimized with low initial dosing and gradual titration. These early adverse effects almost always attenuate after the first few weeks of treatment. Sexual dysfunction (see "Sexual Dysfunction" subsection later in this section) is the most common long-term side effect of SSRIs.

Gastrointestinal Symptoms

Nausea is a common early side effect of all SSRIs. Early nausea is probably attributable to the stimulation of serotonin type 3 (5-HT$_3$) receptors in the gastrointestinal tract, which downregulate after several weeks of treatment. Hence this side effect is both dose dependent and transient. Some patients report less nausea if they take the medication with food. Although rarely needed, medication that blocks the 5-HT$_3$ receptor (e.g., ondansetron) can be used to reduce SSRI-induced nausea.

Sexual Dysfunction

Decreased libido, anorgasmia, and delayed ejaculation are common side effects of SSRIs. When possible, management of sexual side effects should be postponed until the patient has completed an adequate trial of the antidepressant.

When significant sexual dysfunction persists for more than 1 month despite a positive response to treatment, a reduction in the dose should be considered. In some cases, this results in a diminution of the symptoms without loss of therapeutic benefit. However, sometimes there is no therapeutic dose that does not cause sexual side effects. In such cases, two strategies are available: the antidepressant can be replaced with an alternative, or other drugs can be prescribed concomitantly to counteract the side effect. The decision to try a different antidepressant is potentially problematic because an equivalent therapeutic response is not guaranteed. In our experience, switching from one SSRI to another does not tend to decrease sexual side effects. Antidepressants that do not commonly cause sexual dysfunction are bupropion, nefazodone, and mirtazapine. Guidelines for changing antidepressants are presented in "Antidepressant Switching" at the end of this chapter.

Several medications have been suggested as antidotes for the sexual side effects associated with antidepressant therapy. Bupropion, 75 or 150 mg/day, has been added to an SSRI regimen with some success in terms of improving libido (Labbate and Pollack 1994). Sildenafil has been used on an as-needed basis before sexual activity (Fava et al. 1998).

Stimulation and Insomnia

Some patients may experience jitteriness, restlessness, muscle tension, and disturbed sleep. These side effects typically occur early in treatment, before the antidepressant effect. All patients should be informed of the possibility of these side effects and be reassured that if they develop, they tend to be transient. In patients with preexisting anxiety, therapy should be started at low doses, with subsequent titration as tolerated. If overstimulation occurs with this approach, it will be less likely to be severe enough to result in nonadherence with therapy. The short-term use of a benzodiazepine also may help the patient cope with overstimulation in the early stages of treatment until tolerance to this side effect occurs. Despite these common transient stimulating effects, SSRIs are clearly effective in patients with anxiety or agitated depression. Similarly, insomnia that commonly occurs early in treatment may be tolerable if the patient is reassured that the side effect will be transient. Symptomatic, short-term treatment with a hypnotic at bedtime is reasonable.

Bleeding

SSRIs affect serotonin systems throughout the body, including serotonin in platelets. Because platelets cannot synthesize serotonin, this effect tends to decrease platelet aggregation, which may lead to abnormal bleeding. Two large studies have reported an association between use of SSRIs and increased risk of upper gastrointestinal bleeding or other abnormal bleeding (Dalton et al. 2003; de Abajo et al. 1999). This is most commonly manifested as bruising, but the rate of clinically significant bleeding is approximately 3.1 patients per 1,000 treatment years. Therefore, it is prudent for clinicians to be cautious about prescribing SSRIs for patients with other risk factors for bleeding and to educate patients to inform clinicians if they notice any abnormal bleeding or bruising.

Neurological Effects

Tension headaches are common early in treatment and usually can be managed with over-the-counter pain relief preparations. SSRIs may initially worsen migraines but are often effective in reducing the severity and frequency of these headaches (Doughty and Lyle 1995; Manna et al. 1994).

Tremor and akathisia are less common and can be managed with dose reduction or the addition of a β-blocker such as propranolol (10–40 mg). There are isolated case reports of SSRI-related dystonia and increasing reports of SSRI-related exacerbation of Parkinson's disease (Di Rocco et al. 1998; Linazasoro 2000). The advisability of SSRI use in depressed patients with Parkinson's disease remains to be determined. Bupropion and electroconvulsive therapy (ECT) may be reasonable alternatives for these patients.

Sedation

SSRIs may induce sedation in some patients. Altering the time of administration (e.g., having the patient take the medication in the evening rather than the morning) is often not successful.

Weight Gain or Loss

All SSRIs have the potential to cause weight gain in some individuals. In a controlled study, Fava and colleagues (2000) found that paroxetine was associated with greater weight gain than were flu-oxetine and sertraline.

Syndrome of Inappropriate Secretion of Antidiuretic Hormone

Case reports have indicated an association between SSRIs and the syndrome of inappropriate secretion of antidiuretic hormone. Symptoms include lethargy, headache, hyponatremia, increased urinary sodium excretion, and hyperosmotic urine. Acute treatment of this syndrome should consist of discontinuation of the drug as well as restriction of fluid intake. Patients experiencing severe con-fusion, convulsions, or coma should receive intravenous sodium chloride. Elderly persons may be at a higher risk for developing this syndrome.

Serotonin Syndrome

The serotonin syndrome results from excess serotonergic stimula-tion of receptors in both the central nervous system and the periph-ery. This syndrome is often mild, but severe forms (often the result of drug-drug interactions) can be fatal. The syndrome must be iden-tified as rapidly as possible. As recently reviewed by Boyer and Shannon (2005), the most common symptoms are confusion, flush-ing, diaphoresis, tremor, and myoclonic jerks. The patient may have symptoms of the serotonin syndrome in the context of monotherapy with a serotonergic medication, but this scenario is less common than symptoms resulting from use of two or more serotonergic drugs concurrently. Discontinuation of the serotonergic medica-tions is the first step in treatment. The 5-HT$_{2A}$ antagonist cyprohep-tadine can be used if further treatment is warranted, beginning with an oral dose of 12 mg and then administering 2 mg every 2 hours. Although cyproheptadine is available only in oral form, tablets may be crushed, mixed in a suspension, and administered via a nasogas-tric tube. Second-generation antipsychotics, such as olanzapine, have 5-HT$_{2A}$ antagonist activity and also may be considered as an-tidotes. However, efficacy has not been established for any of these presumed antidotes.

Discontinuation Syndrome

Several reports have described a series of symptoms after discontinuation or dose reduction of serotonergic antidepressant medications. The most common symptoms include dizziness, headache, paresthesia, nausea, diarrhea, insomnia, and irritability. Of note, these symptoms may also be seen when a patient misses doses. A prospective, double-blind, placebo-substitution study confirmed that discontinuation symptoms are most common with short half-life antidepressants, such as paroxetine (Rosenbaum et al. 1998).

Apathy Syndrome

We and others have noted an apathy syndrome in some patients after months or years of successful treatment with SSRIs. Patients often confuse this syndrome with a recurrence of depression, but the two conditions are quite distinct. The syndrome is characterized by a loss of motivation, increased passivity, and feelings of lethargy and "flatness." However, sadness, tearfulness, emotional angst, decreased concentration, feelings of hopelessness or worthlessness, and thoughts of suicide are not associated with this syndrome. If specifically asked, patients often remark that the symptoms are not experientially similar to their original depressive symptoms. This syndrome has not been adequately studied, and the pathophysiology is not known. However, there is speculation that subchronic stimulation of central serotonin attenuates dopamine functioning in several areas of the brain, including the frontal cortex. The apathy syndrome appears to be dose dependent and reversible. Mistakenly interpreting the apathy and lethargy as a relapse of depression, and consequently increasing the dose of medication, will lead to worsening of symptoms. If dose reduction is not effective, adding a stimulant may be beneficial (see Chapter 6). Other agents that increase dopamine also may be effective. Olanzapine, which increases frontal lobe dopamine, also has been reported to be effective in the treatment of apathy in patients taking SSRIs (Marangell et al. 2002).

Vivid Dreams

Reports of vivid dreams (not nightmares) are common with SSRI therapy. The mechanism is unknown.

Rash

If a mild rash develops, the drug may be continued and symptomatic treatment instituted. Severe rashes require discontinuation of medication. Because the SSRIs share similar mechanisms but not similar structures, an allergy to one agent does not predict an allergy to another.

Drug Interactions

Several deaths have been reported among patients taking a combination of SSRIs and MAOIs; these deaths were presumably due to the serotonin syndrome. Because of the potential lethality of this interaction, a patient who needs to switch from an SSRI to an MAOI must not begin taking the MAOI until the SSRI has been fully eliminated from his or her body. This time frame is five times the half-life of the SSRI. Therefore, a wait of at least 5 weeks is required between discontinuation of fluoxetine and institution of MAOI therapy, and about 1 week should elapse between use of other SSRIs and initiation of treatment with an MAOI. A 2-week waiting period is required when switching from an MAOI to an SSRI, to allow resynthesis of the monoamine oxidase enzyme. The concurrent use of SSRIs and triptans (e.g., sumatriptan) has been reported to result in symptoms consistent with mild to moderate serotonin syndrome, but most patients tolerate this combination (Gardner and Lynd 1998). SSRIs vary with regard to inhibition of cytochrome P450 enzymes. Enzyme inhibition may result in increased blood levels of concomitantly administered medications that rely on the inhibited enzyme for their metabolism (see Chapter 1).

■ SELECTIVE SEROTONIN-NOREPINEPHRINE REUPTAKE INHIBITORS

Although the SSRIs provided a tremendous advantage over the TCAs in terms of tolerability, an effect on norepinephrine also has some theoretical advantages. For example, some authors have suggested that dual reuptake inhibitors may be more likely to lead to remission (Thase et al. 2001). As the name of the class implies, these agents affect the reuptake of both serotonin and norepinephrine, while having very little effect on muscarinic, histaminic or H_1, or α_1-adrenergic receptors. Hence these medications share many of the tolerability and safety benefits of the SSRIs. Currently, two serotonin-norepinephrine reuptake inhibitors (SNRIs) are available in the United States: venlafaxine and duloxetine.

Venlafaxine   Effexor

Venlafaxine is approved by the U.S. Food and Drug Administration for the treatment of both major depression and generalized anxiety disorder. Preliminary data suggest that it might also have a role in the treatment of chronic pain conditions and perhaps other disorders against which SSRIs are effective. Serotonin reuptake inhibition is prominent at lower doses of venlafaxine; at higher doses, inhibition of norepinephrine reuptake becomes more significant.

Venlafaxine is 27% protein bound; in all other antidepressants, protein binding is substantially greater. This property of venlafaxine is advantageous when it is necessary to minimize the likelihood of protein-binding interactions. Venlafaxine is unlikely to inhibit cytochrome P450 enzymes, and therefore the likelihood of drug interactions is further decreased. Extended-release venlafaxine allows for once-daily dosing. Blood pressure may increase at higher doses (see "Hypertension" subsection later in this section).

Clinical Use

The recommended dose range is 75–225 mg/day. The extended-release preparation, which allows for once-daily dosing in most patients, is preferred over the short-acting preparation. The usual starting dose is 37.5–75 mg/day. Doses up to 375 mg/day have been used in patients who were otherwise nonresponsive to treatment. Blood pressure monitoring is recommended because of dose-dependent increases in mean diastolic blood pressure in some patients.

Unlike SSRIs, venlafaxine shows a positive dose-response relation: patients with mild depression may respond to lower doses, whereas patients with more severe or recurrent depression may respond better to higher doses.

Risks, Side Effects, and Their Management

The side-effect profile of venlafaxine is similar to that of SSRIs and includes gastrointestinal symptoms, sexual dysfunction, and transient discontinuation symptoms. Like the SSRIs, venlafaxine does not affect cardiac conduction or lower the seizure threshold. In most patients, venlafaxine is not associated with sedation or weight gain. Side effects that differ from those of SSRIs are hypothesized to be related to the increased noradrenergic activity of this drug at higher doses; these side effects are dose-dependent anxiety (in some patients) and dose-dependent hypertension.

Hypertension.   Modest dose-dependent increases in blood pressure may occur with venlafaxine treatment. A large meta-analysis found that the magnitude of change in blood pressure associated with venlafaxine use is statistically significant but is unlikely to be of clinical significance at doses less than 300 mg/day (Thase 1998). However, the incidence of hypertension is 13% at dosages greater than 300 mg/day. If clinically significant treatment-emergent hypertension occurs, dose reduction or treatment discontinuation should be considered.

Overdose

Few data are available regarding venlafaxine in overdose, but the drug's pharmacological profile suggests that it is safer than TCAs. In most of the reported cases to date, symptoms were not present.

In other cases, somnolence, mild sinus tachycardia, and generalized convulsions were noted. Recommended treatment includes general supportive and symptomatic measures. In severe cases, dialysis should be considered.

Drug Interactions

Venlafaxine does not appear to inhibit cytochrome P450 enzymes significantly, and it is the antidepressant least likely to contribute to protein-binding interactions. Because of the risk of serotonin syndrome, venlafaxine should not be combined with MAOIs.

Duloxetine

Duloxetine hydrochloride is an SNRI that is approved by the U.S. Food and Drug Administration for the treatment of both major depression and the pain associated with diabetic peripheral neuropathy. Duloxetine affects both serotonin and norepinephrine reuptake inhibition at 60 mg, which is the recommended starting and therapeutic dosage. Interestingly, it does not appear to induce sustained treatment-emergent hypertension compared with placebo, although rare cases are possible. Its half-life is approximately 12 hours, and it is greater than 90% protein bound. The most frequent side effect is early nausea, which is dose dependent and typically transient. Like venlafaxine, duloxetine is weight neutral, meaning that most patients do not gain or lose weight during treatment.

Clinical Use

The recommended dosage for the treatment of major depression is 60 mg/day, whereas in diabetic neuropathy, a dosage of up to 120 mg/day is recommended. Some patients with major depression may experience greater efficacy with dosages of 90 or 120 mg/day. Nausea in the early phases of treatment is dose dependent, so treatment-naive patients might benefit from starting at 30 mg for the first week and then increasing to the target dose of 60 mg. The use of duloxetine to treat primary fibromyalgia is supported by a randomized, double-blind, placebo-controlled trial (Arnold et al. 2004). Note that the dose of duloxetine in this study was 120 mg, similar to that in the neuropathic pain studies.

Risks, Side Effects, and Their Management

The side-effect profile of duloxetine is similar to that of SSRIs. Like the SSRIs, duloxetine does not affect cardiac conduction or lower the seizure threshold. In most patients, duloxetine is not associated with sedation. Side effects that differ from those of SSRIs are hypothesized to be related to the increased noradrenergic activity of this drug and include dry mouth, constipation, and increased sweating.

Nausea.   Patients should be educated that they may experience nausea but that this side effect typically subsides within a week. In clinical trials, only 1.4% of the patients discontinued the medication because of this side effect.

Hepatotoxicity.   Duloxetine is rarely associated with increases in serum transaminase levels, typically in the first 2 months of treatment. In controlled trials in major depressive disorder, elevations of alanine aminotransferase (ALT) to greater than three times the upper limit of normal occurred in 0.9% (8 of 930) of the duloxetine-treated patients and in 0.3% (2 of 652) of the placebo-treated patients. Current product labeling contains a caution regarding the use of duloxetine in patients with significant alcohol use or chronic liver disease. Postmarketing reports have indicated that increases in transaminases have occurred in some patients with chronic liver disease (Cymbalta 2005).

Uncontrolled narrow-angle glaucoma.   In clinical trials, duloxetine use was associated with an increased risk of mydriasis; therefore, it should not be used in patients with uncontrolled narrow-angle glaucoma.

Sexual dysfunction.   The controlled clinical trials of duloxetine in the treatment of major depression used a rating scale to assess prospectively treatment-emergent sexual dysfunction. As with

SSRIs and venlafaxine, males who received duloxetine experienced more difficulty with ability to reach orgasm than did males who received placebo. However, females did not experience more sexual dysfunction while taking duloxetine than did those taking placebo. The reason for fewer sexual side effects in females is not clear, and some females will experience treatment-emergent anorgasmia or decreased libido.

Overdose

Few data are available regarding duloxetine in overdose. Recommended treatment includes general supportive and symptomatic measures. Dialysis is not recommended because the drug is highly protein bound.

Drug Interactions

Duloxetine is a moderate inhibitor of the CYP 2D6 enzyme and may increase the levels of other medications that use this enzyme (Table 1–1). Because of the risk of serotonin syndrome, duloxetine should not be combined with MAOIs. Because duloxetine is highly bound to plasma protein, combination with another drug that is highly protein bound may cause increased free concentrations of the other drug, potentially resulting in adverse events.

■ BUPROPION   Wellbutrin

The most significant advantage of bupropion is its relative lack of sexual side effects. Indeed, the addition of low doses of bupropion may attenuate the sexual dysfunction caused by other medications. Because bupropion facilitates dopamine transmission, many clinicians preferentially use this agent for patients with Parkinson's disease. The fact that dopamine is integrally related to the brain's reward mechanisms, which are stimulated by nicotine and other addictive substances, has provided the theoretical underpinning for recent research indicating that bupropion is an effective aid in smoking cessation. In two placebo-controlled trials involving nondepressed, chronic cigarette smokers, there was a dose-dependent increase in the percentage of patients able to achieve abstinence (Zyban 2005). Individuals receiving 300 mg of bupropion daily were able to sustain abstinence longer than were those receiving 150 mg/day, and results achieved by patients given bupropion were superior to those achieved in the placebo groups. Bupropion is being marketed under the name Zyban as a tool for smoking cessation.

Overall, bupropion has a favorable side-effect profile. The drug is associated with little or no weight gain, has few effects on cardiac conduction, and has minimal sexual side effects. Disadvantages include an increased risk of medication-induced seizures at higher-than-recommended doses.

Clinical Use

Use of the extended-release (XL) preparation is recommended because of increased tolerability, decreased seizure risk, and the increased ease of use associated with a once-a-day preparation. Treatment with the sustained-release (SR) or XL preparation is initiated at a dose of 150 mg, preferably taken in the morning. After 4 days, the dosage may be increased to 150 mg twice a day (SR) or 300 mg once daily in the morning (XL). Gradual dose titration helps to minimize initial anxiety and insomnia. Temporary use of anxiolytic or hypnotic agents is reasonable in some patients but generally should be limited to the first few weeks of treatment.

Contraindications

Patients with seizure disorders should not take bupropion. Similarly, an alternative treatment should be considered in the case of patients with a history of significant head trauma, a central nervous system tumor, or an active eating disorder.

Risks, Side Effects, and Their Management

The most common side effects of bupropion are initial headache, anxiety, insomnia, increased sweating, and gastrointestinal upset.

Tremor and akathisia also may occur. Management is the same as that for SSRI side effects. Bupropion is not associated with anticholinergic side effects, orthostatic hypotension, weight gain, or cardiac conduction changes.

The incidence of seizures with the immediate-release preparation is 0.4% at doses less than 450 mg/day, provided no single dose of the short-acting preparation exceeds 150 mg. The incidence increases to 5% at doses between 450 and 600 mg/day. The SR preparation is associated with seizure incidences of 0.1% at doses less than 300 mg/day and 0.4% at doses between 300 and 400 mg/day. Higher doses of the SR preparation have not been evaluated. No single dose of greater than 200 mg is recommended for the SR preparation, whereas up to 450 mg at a single dose may be given with the XL preparation. Bupropion should be used with caution in patients with a history of seizures or who are taking concomitant medications that lower the seizure threshold.

Psychosis

Reports of delusions, hallucinations, and paranoia are consistent with bupropion-mediated increases in central dopamine. Bupropion should be used with caution in patients with psychotic disorders.

Overdose

Much more is known about overdose with the immediate-release formulation of bupropion than with the newer, SR and XL formulations. Reported reactions to overdose with the immediate-release form include seizures, hallucinations, loss of consciousness, and sinus tachycardia. Treatment of overdose should include induction of vomiting, administration of activated charcoal, and electrocardiographic and electroencephalographic monitoring. For seizures, an intravenous benzodiazepine preparation is recommended.

The danger of bupropion overdose is limited to the risk of seizures for the most part. However, seizures are seldom life threatening unless they result in motor vehicle accidents, falls, or other trauma-related events. Bupropion's lack of significant cardiovascular or respiratory toxicity means that it is rarely lethal in overdose.

Drug Interactions

The combination of bupropion with an MAOI is potentially dangerous, but less so than the combination of serotonergic drugs and MAOIs. Although the practice is not recommended, MAOIs and bupropion have been combined in patients with refractory depression.

In vitro data suggest that bupropion is metabolized by CYP 2B6. Bupropion inhibits CYP 2D6. Because of the risk of dose-dependent seizures, caution is warranted when bupropion is combined with other medications that might inhibit its metabolism.

■ NEFAZODONE Serzone

Nefazodone is primarily a postsynaptic 5-HT$_2$ antagonist. Nefazodone continues to be available in generic formulations, mostly for patients who have been stabilized previously while taking this medication and need ongoing treatment. The branded product was removed from the market in 2003 subsequent to reports of hepatotoxicity. The reported rate of liver failure resulting in death or transplant in the United States is approximately 1 case per 250,000–300,000 patient-years of exposure (Serzone 2002). Patients taking nefazodone whose condition is currently stable may wish to continue this treatment rather than switch to an alternative agent because nefazodone does not appear to cause weight gain or sexual dysfunction. Individuals who develop increased serum transaminase levels of three times the upper limits of the normal range or higher should be withdrawn from nefazodone and not be considered for rechallenge.

Drug Interactions

Coadministration with most medications that are metabolized by CYP 3A3/4 should be undertaken with caution, and the doses of the other medications that are CYP 3A3/4 substrates (see Table 1–1) should be reduced. The interaction between nefazodone and MAOIs has not yet been evaluated, but it may be as dangerous as the interaction between SSRIs and MAOIs. Therefore, combining nefazodone and MAOIs should be avoided.

■ TRAZODONE *Desyrel*

Trazodone is an older antidepressant that is associated with significant sedation. Currently, trazodone is not recommended as a first-line antidepressant because of an increased risk of orthostatic hypotension, arrhythmias, and priapism. Also, compared with other available antidepressants, trazodone does not offer an advantage in terms of therapeutic efficacy. However, trazodone may be useful in patients with insomnia. It is currently common practice to use low doses of trazodone (e.g., 50–100 mg) to assist with initial insomnia while starting treatment with one of the newer antidepressants to address the underlying depression. If this strategy is used, we recommend tapering the trazodone dose and discontinuing treatment with trazodone after 4–6 weeks.

Risks, Side Effects, and Their Management

Excessive sedation is the most commonly encountered side effect of trazodone. Although trazodone has virtually no anticholinergic side effects, dry mouth and blurred vision occur more frequently with trazodone treatment than with placebo.

Priapism

Trazodone is the only antidepressant that has been associated with priapism, which may be irreversible and require surgical intervention.

Overdose

Trazodone overdose carries a risk of myocardial irritation in patients with preexisting ventricular conduction abnormalities.

■ MIRTAZAPINE *Remeron*

Mirtazapine has been shown to reduce anxiety symptoms and sleep disturbances associated with depression, as early as 1 week after the start of treatment. Other advantages are minimal sexual dysfunction, minimal nausea, and once-daily dosing. In addition, mirtazapine is unlikely to be associated with cytochrome P450–mediated drug interactions. The disadvantages of mirtazapine are weight gain and prominent early sedation.

Clinical Use

Mirtazapine treatment is initiated at a dosage of 15 mg qhs. Depending on clinical response and side effects, the dosage can be increased to a maximum of 45 mg at bedtime, although higher doses are sometimes used in treatment-resistant patients. Elderly patients and individuals with renal or hepatic disease may require lower doses.

Risks, Side Effects, and Their Management

As noted previously, sexual dysfunction and nausea are not commonly associated with mirtazapine treatment. The most common side effects are sedation, weight gain, and dizziness.

Somnolence

Somnolence occurs in more than 50% of the patients taking mirtazapine. Tolerance to this side effect develops after the first few weeks of treatment. Higher doses do not appear to produce significantly greater sedation.

Weight Gain

The weight gain associated with mirtazapine use may be partially caused by increased appetite. A mean increase of 3.7 kg over the first 28 weeks of treatment has been reported in several controlled studies (Bremner 1995; Smith et al. 1990). More recently, a relapse-prevention study with 410 depressed patients taking mirtazapine reported a mean increase in body weight of 2.5 kg after 12 weeks and a mean increase in body weight of 3.3 kg after 40 weeks (Thase et al. 2000).

Agranulocytosis

In preliminary clinical trials, 2 of 2,796 mirtazapine-treated patients developed agranulocytosis, and 1 developed severe neutropenia. All 3 patients recovered after medication discontinuation, and other possible etiologies were present in at least 1 of these individuals. Thirteen patients with pretreatment neutropenia did develop more severe neutropenia or agranulocytosis. Postmarketing evaluation to date has not established a causal relation between mirtazapine and agranulocytosis. Routine laboratory monitoring is not currently recommended.

Anticholinergic Effects

Mirtazapine is associated with modest anticholinergic side effects, including dry mouth and constipation. Anticholinergic side effects and their management are discussed in the "Tricyclic and Heterocyclic Antidepressants" section later in this chapter.

Cardiovascular Effects

Hypertension, orthostatic hypotension, dizziness, and vasodilation with peripheral edema may occur with mirtazapine treatment.

Overdose

Little is known about mirtazapine overdose. To date, patients who have overdosed have fully recovered. Warning signs include drowsiness, impaired memory, and tachycardia. Recommended treatment includes gastric lavage, cardiac monitoring, and supportive measures.

Drug Interactions

Mirtazapine does not significantly inhibit hepatic cytochrome P450 enzymes. Additive effects may occur when mirtazapine is combined with other drugs with sedative or vascular effects. Mirtazapine should not be used in combination with an MAOI or within 14 days of discontinuing treatment with an MAOI. When it is combined with fluvoxamine, a potent inhibitor of P450 enzymes—including 1A2, 2D6, and 3A4, which metabolizes mirtazapine—the plasma concentration of mirtazapine may be increased by up to fourfold (Anttila et al. 2001; Demers et al. 2001).

■ TRICYCLIC AND HETEROCYCLIC ANTIDEPRESSANTS

TCAs derive their name from their chemical structure; all tricyclics have a three-ring nucleus. Currently, most clinicians are moving away from using TCAs as first-line drugs; relative to the newer antidepressants, they tend to have more side effects, to require gradual titration to achieve an adequate antidepressant dose, and to be lethal in overdose. Some data suggest that TCAs may be more effective than SSRIs in the treatment of major depression with melancholic features (Danish University Antidepressant Group 1990; Perry 1996), however, many skilled clinicians and researchers continue to prefer the newer antidepressants, even for patients with melancholia, for the aforementioned reasons. Newer medications that affect both norepinephrine and serotonin (e.g., venlafaxine and mirtazapine) also may have superior efficacy in severely ill depressed patients or when remission is defined as the outcome (Thase et al. 2001).

Imipramine, amitriptyline, clomipramine, trimipramine, and doxepin are tertiary amine TCAs. Desipramine, nortriptyline, and protriptyline are secondary amine TCAs. Tertiary amine tricyclics have more potent serotonin reuptake inhibition, and secondary amine tricyclics have more potent noradrenergic reuptake inhibition. Tertiary amine TCAs tend to have more side effects than do secondary amine TCAs. Desipramine and protriptyline tend to be activating. Among the TCAs, nortriptyline is the least likely to produce orthostatic hypotension. Because amoxapine has an active metabolite that antagonizes dopamine D_2 receptors, it can cause treatment-emergent extrapyramidal side effects (see Chapter 4).

Clinical Use

In the case of patients with preexisting heart disease and patients older than 40 years, an electrocardiogram should be obtained before the initiation of TCA treatment. TCAs should not be used in patients with bundle branch block unless all other options have failed.

The following dose guidelines are for healthy adults with minimal anxiety. Patients with significant anxiety, panic, or a tendency to be sensitive to side effects should receive initial doses that are 50% lower. Similarly, elderly patients and patients with cardiovascular or hepatic disease should receive lower initial doses.

Imipramine, amitriptyline, doxepin, desipramine, clomipramine, and trimipramine therapy can be initiated at 25–50 mg/day. Divided dosing may be used at first to minimize side effects, but eventually the entire dose can be given at bedtime. The dose can be increased to 150 mg/day the second week, 225 mg/day the third week, and 300 mg/ day the fourth week. The dose of clomipramine should not exceed 250 mg/day because of an increased risk of seizures at higher doses.

Nortriptyline therapy should be initiated at 25 mg/day, and the dose should be increased to 75 mg/day over 1–2 weeks depending on tolerability and clinical response. Some patients require doses of up to 150 mg/day. Amoxapine therapy should be started at 50 mg/day, and the dose should be titrated to 400 mg/day; amoxapine has a short half-life and should be given in divided doses. Treatment with protriptyline can be started at 10 mg/day, and the dose can be increased to up to 60 mg/day. Maprotiline therapy should be started at 50 mg/day, and that dose should be maintained for 2 weeks; the risk of seizure is increased if the dose is raised too quickly. The dose can be increased over 4 weeks to 225 mg/day.

Plasma Levels and Therapeutic Monitoring

Clinically meaningful plasma levels are available for imipramine, desipramine, and nortriptyline. For imipramine, the sum of the plasma levels of imipramine and the desmethyl metabolite (desipramine) should be greater than 200–250 ng/mL. Desipramine levels should be greater than 125 ng/mL. A therapeutic window has been noted for nortriptyline, with optimal response between 50 and 150 ng/mL. These therapeutic levels are based on steady-state concentrations, which are reached after 5–7 days of administration of these medications. Blood should be drawn approximately 10–14 hours after the last dose of medication.

Risks, Side Effects, and Their Management

Anticholinergic Effects

Anticholinergic side effects result from antagonism of muscarinic receptors. The most common anticholinergic side effects are dry mouth, constipation, urinary retention, blurred vision, and tachycardia. In predisposed patients, such as elderly persons, anticholinergic medications may cause cognitive impairment and confusion. Because the tertiary amines and protriptyline have a particularly high affinity for muscarinic receptors, these medications are more likely than others to have anticholinergic side effects.

Cholinergic medications (e.g., bethanechol chloride) have been reported to relieve some of the anticholinergic side effects. The addition of a medication to treat side effects should be considered only after dose reduction and alternative antidepressants with fewer anticholinergic side effects have been tried. One must proceed with great caution when using antidepressants with anticholinergic side effects in treating patients with prostatic hypertrophy, narrow-angle glaucoma, or cognitive impairment. The newer antidepressant drugs may be preferable for patients with these disorders. Pilocarpine oral rinse or eyedrops can be helpful for local relief of symptoms.

Sedation

The relative sedating properties of TCAs appear to parallel their respective histamine receptor binding affinities. Trimipramine, amitriptyline, and doxepin are the most sedating TCAs. Desipramine and protriptyline are less sedating.

Cardiovascular Effects

Cardiovascular effects include orthostatic hypotension, tachycardia, and cardiac conduction delays. Although TCAs at toxic levels (as occur in overdose) can cause life-threatening arrhythmias, TCAs are potent antiarrhythmic agents, possessing quinidine-like properties (Glassman and Bigger 1981). Because prolongation of PR and QRS intervals can occur with TCA use, these drugs should not be used in patients with preexisting heart block (especially right bundle branch block and left bundle branch block). In such patients, treatment with TCAs often leads to second- or third-degree heart block, both life-threatening conditions. Orthostatic hypotension may not be dose dependent.

Weight Gain

Weight gain is a common side effect. Secondary amines are less likely than tertiary amines to produce weight gain.

Seizures

A dose-related risk of seizures has been found with clomipramine, which has led to the recommendation that the total daily dose of this drug not exceed 250 mg. Overdoses of TCAs, particularly amoxapine and desipramine, are associated with seizures. Whether therapeutic doses of TCAs lower the seizure threshold is controversial. Nonetheless, other classes may be safer options for individuals with epilepsy.

Extrapyramidal Side Effects (Amoxapine Only)

Amoxapine, which has a mild neuroleptic effect, can cause extrapyramidal side effects, akathisia, and even tardive dyskinesia.

Overdose

The major complications of TCA overdose include those that arise from neuropsychiatric impairment, hypotension, cardiac arrhythmias, and seizures. Because TCAs have significant anticholinergic activity, anticholinergic delirium may occur. Other complications of anticholinergic overdose include agitation, supraventricular arrhythmias, hallucinations, severe hypertension, and seizures. Patients with anticholinergic delirium have hot, dry skin; dry mucous membranes; dilated pupils; absent bowel sounds; and tachycardia. Anticholinergic delirium constitutes a medical emergency and requires full supportive medical care. Physostigmine, a centrally and peripherally acting reversible acetylcholinesterase inhibitor, may be used as a diagnostic agent in cases of suspected anticholinergic toxicity. This agent is administered intramuscularly at a dose of 1–2 mg, or intravenously at a slow, controlled rate of no more than 1 mg/minute. Physostigmine should not be used to maintain reversal of the toxicity, however, because a cholinergic crisis may result. A cholinergic crisis is characterized by nausea, vomiting, bradycardia, and seizures. This reaction can be reversed by administering a potent anticholinergic drug such as atropine.

Hypotension, which may result from norepinephrine depletion or have other causes related to peripheral and central effects of TCAs, should be treated with vigorous fluid replacement. Seizures and cardiac complications also may occur with antidepressant overdose. When the QRS interval is less than 0.10 second, the likelihood of seizures or ventricular arrhythmias decreases (Boehnert and Lovejoy 1985). Ventricular arrhythmias that occur secondary to overdose are typical of arrhythmias resulting from high doses of quinidine-like agents and begin within the first 24 hours after hospital admission (Goldberg et al. 1985). Ventricular arrhythmias should be treated with lidocaine, propranolol, or phenytoin. Prophylactic treatment with phenytoin and insertion of a temporary pacemaker should be considered in patients with prolonged QRS intervals (i.e., longer than 120 ms).

Drug Interactions

Because the liver metabolizes TCAs, drugs that inhibit or induce hepatic microsomal enzymes may alter plasma tricyclic levels. This is particularly true of CYP 2D6 inhibitors. In some individuals, this interaction may result in dangerously high levels of the TCA when a potent 2D6 inhibitor, such as paroxetine, is coadministered.

Although several agents affect tricyclic levels, the effect is usually not reciprocal; TCAs rarely affect the metabolism of other drugs. A notable exception to this general rule is valproate sodium, levels of which may decrease when a TCA is administered concurrently. By a different mode of action, TCAs also may interfere with the mechanism of action of two antihypertensive drugs. Both guanethidine and clonidine lose effectiveness if administered concomitantly with drugs (such as TCAs) that block reuptake of catecholamines into adrenergic neurons.

■ MONOAMINE OXIDASE INHIBITORS

Because of the improved tolerability and safety of newer antidepressants, MAOIs are not currently used as first-line agents. However, MAOIs remain excellent medications for patients whose symptoms do not respond to the newer antidepressant drugs. Patients with atypical depression, characterized by oversleeping and overeating, show a preferential response to MAOI therapy compared with TCAs (Liebowitz et al. 1984; Quitkin et al. 1979; Ravaris et al. 1980; Zisook 1985).

Monoamine oxidase A (MAO A) acts selectively on the substrates norepinephrine and serotonin, whereas monoamine oxidase B (MAO B) preferentially affects phenylethylamine. Both MAO A and MAO B oxidize dopamine and tyramine. MAO A inhibition appears to be most relevant to the antidepressant effects of these drugs. Drugs that inhibit both MAO A and MAO B are called *nonselective*. The MAOI antidepressants currently available in the United States are nonselective inhibitors. Because tyramine can be metabolized by either MAO A or MAO B, drugs that selectively inhibit one of these enzymes but not the other do not require dietary

TABLE 2–4.   **MAOI reversibility and selectivity**

Drug	Reversible inhibition	Enzyme selectivity	Indication
Isocarboxazid	No	MAO A+B	Depression
Phenelzine	No	MAO A+B	Depression
Tranylcypromine	No	MAO A+B	Depression
Selegiline	No	MAO B[a]	Parkinson's disease
Pargyline	No	MAO B[a]	Hypertension
Moclobemide[b]	Yes	MAO A	Depression

Note.   MAOI=monoamine oxidase inhibitor; MAO=monoamine oxidase.
[a]Selective at lower doses, nonselective at higher doses.
[b]Not available in the United States.

restrictions. MAO A–selective drugs, such as moclobemide, are available in other countries (e.g., Canada) for the treatment of depression. MAO B–selective drugs, such as pargyline and selegiline (L-deprenyl), are marketed for other indications and do not appear to treat depression when administered at their usual doses. At higher doses, pargyline and selegiline become nonselective.

Another important characteristic of MAOIs is the production of reversible versus irreversible enzyme inhibition. An irreversible inhibitor permanently disables the enzyme. This means that MAO must be resynthesized, in the absence of the drug, before the activity of the enzyme can be reestablished. Resynthesis of the enzyme may take up to 2 weeks. For this reason, an interval of 10–14 days is required after discontinuing irreversible inhibitors and before instituting treatment with other antidepressants or permitting the use of contraindicated drugs or the consumption of contraindicated foods. On the other hand, a reversible inhibitor can move away from the active site of the enzyme, making the enzyme available to metabolize other substances. The reversibility and selectivity of the currently available MAOIs are summarized in Table 2–4.

Clinical Use

More so than with other medications, it is imperative to review the patient's medical status and current medications before pre-

TABLE 2–5.   Dietary and medication restrictions for patients taking nonselective MAOIs

Foods to avoid while taking an MAOI and for 2 weeks after discontinuing the medication

Aged cheeses

Aged or fermented meats (e.g., sausage, salami, pepperoni)

All foods that may be spoiled

Fava beans and broad bean pods

Meat extracts (e.g., Bovril)

Sauerkraut

Soy sauce

Tap beer, including nonalcoholic tap beer

Yeast extracts (e.g., Marmite)

Safe foods

Alcohol (but not tap beer), in moderation

Fresh cheeses (e.g., cream cheese, cottage cheese, ricotta cheese, American cheese, moderate amounts of mozzarella)

Fresh yogurt

Smoked salmon and whitefish

Yeast and baked goods containing yeast

TABLE 2–5. Dietary and medication restrictions for patients taking nonselective MAOIs (*continued*)

Drugs to avoid while taking an MAOI and for 2 weeks after discontinuing the medication

All sympathomimetic and stimulant drugs, including:

Amphetamines	Local anesthetic drugs containing epinephrine or cocaine
Buspirone	Meperidine
Diet medications	Methylphenidate
Ephedrine	Other antidepressant medications
Fenfluramine and dexfenfluramine	Phenylephrine
Isoproterenol	Phenylpropanolamine
Levodopa and dopamine	

Over-the-counter nasal decongestants; cold, sinus, and allergy medications containing pseudoephedrine, phenylephrine, or phenylpropanolamine; and supplements:

Actifed	NyQuil
Alka-Seltzer Plus	Robitussin PE, DM, CF, Night Relief
Allerest	Sine-Aid
Contac	Sine-Off
Coricidin D	Sinex
CoTylenol	St. John's wort
Dristan	Triaminic
L-tryptophan	Tylenol
Neo-Synephrine	Vicks 44M, 44D

TABLE 2–5. Dietary and medication restrictions for patients taking nonselective MAOIs *(continued)*

Safe cold and allergy medications

Alka-Seltzer (plain)

Chlor-Trimeton Allergy (without decongestant)

Robitussin (plain)

Steroid inhalers

Tylenol (plain)

Other safe medications

Antibiotics

Codeine

Laxatives and stool softeners

Local anesthetics without epinephrine or cocaine

Morphine

Nonsteroidal anti-inflammatory drugs

Note.   MAOI=monoamine oxidase inhibitor.

scribing an MAOI. The importance of complying with dietary and medication restrictions, outlined in Table 2–5, should be discussed with the patient when nonselective MAOIs are being used. The discussion should be supplemented with written instructions, as presented in Table 2–6. Currently, nonselective MAOIs are used predominantly in patients with refractory depression—patients who are often suicidal. Too often, clinicians are hesitant to prescribe MAOIs in such cases because they fear that these patients will intentionally not comply with dietary restrictions, in order to harm themselves. This is a paradox; if the medication is effective, the patient will no longer want to commit suicide. Furthermore, withholding effective treatment, an action that will likely result in continuation of the depressed state, is associated with a higher risk of suicide. In these cases, we often emphasize to the patient that failure to comply with restrictions is more likely to cause cerebral hemorrhage and disability than to cause death.

Phenelzine therapy is initiated at a dose of 15 mg in the morning, and the dose is increased by 15 mg every other day until a total daily dose of 60 mg is reached. If no response occurs within 2 weeks, the dose may be increased in 15-mg increments to a usual maximum of 90 mg/day. Higher doses are sometimes used, if tolerated, in patients with severe, refractory depression. Treatment with tranylcypromine is initiated at a dose of 10 mg, and the dose is then increased every other day to 30 mg/day. As with phenelzine, higher doses may be necessary when the condition is refractory to treatment (Amsterdam and Berwish 1989). After tolerance to the hypotensive side effects has developed, usually after 1 or 2 weeks, the patient may take the medication in a single daily dose in the morning. Morning dosing is preferred because these medications tend to be activating; this is especially true of tranylcypromine, which is related to amphetamine. The typical starting dose of moclobemide is 100 mg three times a day. Higher doses may improve efficacy. The maximum recommended dosage is 600 mg/day, but many clinicians use higher dosages.

| TABLE 2–6. | **Instructions for patients taking nonselective monoamine oxidase inhibitors** |

Avoid all foods and drugs on the list (see Table 2–5).

In general, all foods you should avoid are decayed, fermented, or aged in some way. Avoid any spoiled food, even if it is not on the list.

If you get a cold or the flu, you may take aspirin or Tylenol. For a cough, glycerin cough drops or cough syrup without dextromethorphan may be used.

All laxatives and stool softeners may be used.

For infections, all antibiotics (such as penicillin, tetracycline, or erythromycin) may be safely prescribed.

Do not take any other medications without first checking with me. These medications include over-the-counter medicines bought without prescription, such as cold tablets, nose drops, cough medicine, and diet pills.

Eating one of the restricted foods may suddenly increase your blood pressure. If this occurs, you will get an explosive headache, particularly in the back of your head and in your temples. Your head and face will feel flushed and full, your heart may pound, and you may perspire heavily and feel nauseated. If this rare reaction occurs, do not lie down because this increases your blood pressure further. If your blood pressure is high, go to the nearest emergency center for evaluation and treatment. Do not wait for a returned telephone call from our office.

If you need medical or dental care while taking this medication, show these restrictions and instructions to the doctor or dentist. Have the doctor or dentist call my office if he or she has any questions or needs further clarification or information.

Side effects such as postural light-headedness, constipation, delay in urination, delay in ejaculation and orgasm, muscle twitching, sedation, fluid retention, insomnia, and excessive sweating are quite common. Many of these side effects lessen after the third week.

Light-headedness may occur after sudden changes in position. It can be avoided by getting up slowly. Taking the tablets with meals lessens this and other side effects.

The medication is rarely effective in less than 3 weeks.

Care should be taken while operating any machinery or driving; some patients have episodes of sleepiness in the early phase of treatment.

Take the medication precisely as directed. Do not change the number of pills without first consulting me.

In spite of the side effects and special dietary restrictions, your medication (a monoamine oxidase inhibitor) is safe and effective when taken as directed.

If any special problems arise, call me at my office.

Source. Adapted from Jenike 1987.

Risks, Side Effects, and Their Management

The following side effects apply to the irreversible, nonselective MAOI antidepressants (phenelzine and tranylcypromine). The most common side effects are orthostatic hypotension, headache, insomnia, weight gain, sexual dysfunction, peripheral edema, and afternoon somnolence. Although MAOIs do not have significant affinity for muscarinic receptors, anticholinergic-like side effects are present at the beginning of treatment. Dry mouth is common but not as marked as in TCA therapy. Fortunately, the more serious side effects, such as hypertensive crisis and serotonin syndrome, are not common.

Hypertensive Crisis

Inactivation of intestinal MAO impairs the metabolism of tyramine. Tyramine can act as a false transmitter and displace norepinephrine from presynaptic storage granules. Therefore, large amounts of dietary tyramine can result in a hypertensive crisis in patients taking MAOIs, because increased amounts of norepinephrine are displaced from adrenergic terminals, resulting in profound α-adrenergic activation. This reaction has also been called the "cheese reaction" because tyramine is present in relatively high concentrations in aged cheese.

Tyramine is formed in foods by the decarboxylation of tyrosine during the aging, ripening, or decaying process of foods. Patients receiving MAOIs should be instructed to avoid the foods listed in Table 2–5. The key foods to avoid are aged cheeses, fermented sausage, sauerkraut, soy sauce, yeast extracts such as Marmite, fava beans and broad beans (which contain dopamine), and any foods that are overripe or spoiled. Fresh, unaged cheeses—such as cottage cheese, ricotta, and cream cheese—are safe. Several foods that were formerly considered dangerous are no longer on the list of prohibited substances. For example, domestic bottled or canned beer is now considered safe when consumed in moderation (Gardner et al. 1996). Most wines and liquors are also considered safe when drunk in moderation. Liver, if fresh, is also probably safe, and caffeine and chocolate are of concern only when consumed in large amounts.

Some drugs with sympathomimetic activity, including certain decongestants and cough syrups, should be avoided because they may precipitate a hypertensive crisis (Table 2–5). However, pure antihistaminic drugs, such as diphenhydramine, and pure expectorants without dextromethorphan, such as guaifenesin, are permissible.

Unfortunately, even perfect compliance with dietary and other restrictions does not guarantee complete protection from MAOI-induced hypertensive crises. There are reports of spontaneous hypertension associated with MAOI therapy. Most of these involved the use of tranylcypromine, but phenelzine also has been implicated.

These reactions range from mild to severe. A patient with a mild reaction may complain of sweating, palpitations, and a slight headache. The most severe reaction manifests as a hypertensive crisis, with severe headache, increased blood pressure, and possible intracerebral hemorrhage. When a patient who is taking an MAOI develops a headache, he or she can use a blood pressure cuff at home to determine whether a true hypertensive crisis might be occurring.

If a patient's blood pressure is greatly increased, pharmacological treatment should be instituted. Treatments for MAOI-induced hypertension include administration of the calcium channel blocker nifedipine and use of drugs with α-adrenergic-blocking properties, such as phentolamine (5 mg intravenous). Because treatment with phentolamine may be associated with cardiac arrhythmias or severe hypotension, this approach should be carried out only in an emergency department setting.

Patients taking MAOIs are advised to carry identification cards that indicate that they are taking MAOIs. Before accepting any medication or anesthetic, patients should notify their physicians that they are taking MAOIs. When patients undergo dental procedures, local anesthetics without vasoconstrictors (e.g., epinephrine) must be used.

Serotonin Syndrome

The combination of serotonergic drugs, such as SSRIs, with MAOIs can result in a potentially fatal hypermetabolic reaction, often referred to as the *serotonin syndrome*. Affected individuals experience lethargy, restlessness, confusion, flushing, diaphoresis, tremor, and myoclonic jerks. As the condition progresses, hyperthermia, hypertonicity, myoclonus, and death may occur. The syndrome must be identified as rapidly as possible. Discontinuation of the serotonergic medications is the first step in treatment, followed by emergency medical treatment as required.

The combination of MAOIs with meperidine, and perhaps with other phenylpiperidine analgesics, also has been implicated in fatal reactions attributed to the serotonin syndrome. Aspirin, nonsteroidal anti-inflammatory drugs, and acetaminophen should be used for mild to moderate pain. Of the narcotic agents, codeine and morphine are safe in combination with MAOIs, although doses may need to be lower than usual.

Cardiovascular Effects

The MAOIs cause significant hypotension, which is often the dose-limiting side effect of these drugs. Expansion of intravascular volume through administration of salt tablets or fludrocortisone may be an effective treatment.

Weight Gain

MAOIs are associated with a risk of significant weight gain during treatment. This side effect appears to occur less frequently with tranylcypromine therapy than with phenelzine treatment.

Sexual Dysfunction

MAOIs are commonly associated with treatment-emergent sexual dysfunction, including decreased libido, delayed ejaculation, anorgasmia, and impotence. Some patients become tolerant to this side effect over time, but more often the problem persists unless the dose is reduced or another medication is used to counter the sexual side effects. The treatment of sexual side effects is discussed in the "Selective Serotonin Reuptake Inhibitors" section earlier in this chapter.

Central Nervous System Effects

Headache and insomnia are common initial side effects that usually disappear after the first few weeks of treatment.

Overdose

MAOIs fall between TCAs and SSRIs in terms of lethality in overdose. Most complications related to MAOI overdose arise from the drugs' stimulation of the sympathetic nervous system. MAOIs are most dangerous when patients experience hypertensive crises as the result of ingesting foods with high tyramine content.

Drug Interactions

Inhibition of MAO can cause severe interactions with other drugs, as detailed in the "Hypertensive Crisis" and "Serotonin Syndrome" subsections earlier in this section. A list of drugs that interact with the nonselective MAOIs is provided in Table 2–5.

■ TREATMENT OF SPECIFIC DISORDERS

Acute Major Depression

In patients receiving antidepressants for acute major depression, the initial therapeutic response is often delayed by several weeks. Patients with severe anxiety or insomnia may benefit from the concurrent, time-limited use of a benzodiazepine or short-acting hypnotic (Chapter 3). A patient may initially experience a return of energy and motivation while still having feelings of hopelessness and excessive guilt. Such patients may be at an increased risk for suicide because a return of energy in an extremely dysphoric individual may provide the impetus and means for an act of self-destruction.

It is a clinical challenge to distinguish symptoms of the illness from medication side effects. Many symptoms that patients attribute to antidepressant treatment—such as constipation, poor memory or concentration, nausea or vomiting, diarrhea, difficulty sitting still, drowsiness, difficulty with urination, palpitations, urinary frequency, and tremors—may be attributable to the illness rather than to the medication. A significant part of treating major depression is encouraging patients to continue treatment despite their perceptions of early medication side effects. It is important to inform patients that more troublesome antidepressant side effects subside after the first 2 weeks of treatment.

An adequate trial of antidepressant medication is defined as treatment with therapeutic doses of a drug for a total of 4 weeks. After 4 weeks of antidepressant treatment, patients can be divided into three groups: those who have achieved a full response, those who have achieved a partial response, and those who have not responded. In the case of patients who achieve full remission, treatment should continue for a minimum of 4–6 months, or longer if the patient has a history of recurrent depression (see "Maintenance Treatment of Major Depression" later in this chapter). If a partial response has been achieved by 4 weeks, a full response may be evident within an additional 2 weeks without further intervention. If the symptoms do not respond at all, the dose should be increased, a different antidepressant should be used, or the therapy should be augmented with another medication (see "Treatment-Resistant Depression" later in this chapter).

Depression With Psychotic Features

Psychotic depression has been reported to respond to combined treatment with antidepressants and antipsychotics; patients with psychotic depression also show a dramatic response to ECT, which is often the treatment of choice for this disorder. Long-term treatment with antipsychotic medications is generally not warranted, but prophylactic antidepressant medication must be continued as in nonpsychotic depression.

Bipolar Depression

A history of episodes of mania or hypomania should suggest the diagnosis of bipolar disorder. Because antidepressants can precipitate manic episodes and increase cycling in bipolar patients (Wehr and Goodwin 1979), use of mood stabilizers (e.g., lithium or lamotrigine) is the appropriate first step in the treatment of bipolar depression (see Chapter 5).

Maintenance Treatment of Major Depression

Results of a National Institute of Mental Health collaborative study indicated that antidepressant therapy should not be discontinued before 4–5 symptom-free months have passed (Prien and Kupfer 1986). Most clinicians treat single episodes of depression for a minimum of 6 months. In most cases, antidepressant medication should be continued at the same dose that resulted in remission—hence the saying, "what gets you well keeps you well."

Unfortunately, depression is often recurrent. After one episode of depression, there is a 50% chance that the patient will have a second episode; after three episodes, there is a 90% chance of recurrence (Depression Guideline Panel 1993). Therefore, longer periods of antidepressant treatment, often called maintenance treatment, are warranted to protect against recurrence (American Psychiatric Association 2000). The value of maintenance antidepressant treatment, with and without psychotherapy, for patients with recurrent depression was established by Frank et al. (1990) in a four-arm, double-blind, placebo-controlled trial. Current World Health Organization guidelines recommend maintenance treatment for patients who have had two or more episodes of major depression within a 5-year period (Coppen et al. 1986). For patients with recurrent depression, prophylaxis treatment is recommended for at least 5 years (Kupfer 1993). Maintenance therapy should be considered for patients with three or more episodes of major depression or those with two or more episodes and a family history of mood disorder, as well as those with a rapid recurrence of depressive episodes, an older age at onset, or severe episodes (Keller 2001). The maintenance regimen should consist of the same dose of the same drug to which the patient initially responded and should last as long as two episode cycles, which at times can be up to 4 or 5 years (Keller 2001). Some patients may require lifelong antidepressant maintenance treatment.

Treatment-Resistant Depression

Patients whose depression has apparently been resistant to standard antidepressant treatment often have had inadequate trials of antidepressants or have been nonadherent with drug therapy. Depression in a patient who has failed to complete an adequate trial of an antidepressant drug does not constitute treatment-resistant depression. A patient who reports a history of robust but short-lived responses to several antidepressants may be manifesting a medication-induced rapid-cycling course. Mild episodes of hypomania during the course of treatment may be overlooked, especially in a productive patient with a high level of functioning and a premorbid history of hyperthymic personality, defined as a chronic state of mild hypomania. In these cases, treatment with a mood stabilizer is indicated (see Chapter 5).

For patients who achieve a true nonresponse or only a partial response, treatment options include switching to another antidepressant and using an augmentation or a combination strategy. Augmentation involves adding another agent that is not an antidepressant, such as lithium, a thyroid hormone, or a psychostimulant. In combination treatment, two antidepressants with different mechanisms of action are combined to produce synergistic effects. Whether to switch, augment, or combine depends on many factors, including the severity of the illness, side effects of the current medication, and the patient's willingness to take more than one medication. For example, when a patient's illness significantly interferes with daily function, augmentation or combination should be considered if the current antidepressant is well tolerated, because such an approach may result in a quicker response. However, a patient with a milder illness who is experiencing significant side effects from the current medication and who is generally uneasy about taking medication will probably be better off if the current medication is switched to a different, single antidepressant.

Of the augmentation strategies, lithium augmentation has the best evidence from randomized controlled trials. However, most of these studies focused on TCAs. We typically start with lithium 600 mg at bedtime. If no response is seen after 2 weeks, the dose should be increased as tolerated. Thyroid supplementation (triiodothyronine) has a 50% response rate, comparable to lithium therapy in a controlled clinical trial (Joffe et al. 1993). For reasons that are unclear, triiodothyronine is apparently more effective than thyroxine as an augmenting agent in unipolar depression (Joffe and Singer 1990).

Stimulants such as amphetamine and methylphenidate have been used to treat depression for many years. Stimulants should not be used alone, except perhaps in geriatric patients with prominent apathy, medically ill patients with depression, or patients with post-stroke depression (Lingam et al. 1988). However, psychostimulants are useful for augmentation of antidepressant therapy in refractory depression, and they are generally safe, even for most patients with cardiac disorders. The nonamphetamine stimulant modafinil was found to be helpful in a recent placebo-controlled study involving 311 patients with partial response to SSRIs (Fava et al. 2005).

The use of more than one antidepressant in patients with treatment-resistant depression is potentially beneficial. SSRI-TCA combinations have been reported to be effective in patients who fail to respond to monotherapy, and the combinations may have a more rapid antidepressant effect. Some SSRIs can cause tricyclic levels in the blood to increase, but this effect is not likely to account for the synergism between the two antidepressants. However, because of this pharmacokinetic interaction, the TCA dose should be reduced to achieve the same blood levels when this combination is used. Although there are few systematic data, other antidepressant combinations are commonly used in clinical practice to treat refractory depression. The key to combining two antidepressants is to choose agents that have different mechanisms of action. For example, it makes little sense to combine two SSRIs, but combining an SSRI with mirtazapine or bupropion may be beneficial. When combining antidepressants, it is important both to ensure that the patient has had an adequate trial of a single agent and to be aware of possible drug interactions or additive side effects. Nonpharmacological options (e.g., ECT, vagus nerve stimulation, and psychotherapy) also should be considered in cases of inadequate response to treatment.

Borderline Personality Disorder

Numerous studies have investigated the treatment of borderline personality disorder with various antidepressants, including TCAs, MAOIs, SSRIs, and venlafaxine (American Psychiatric Association 2001; Soloff 2000). The American Psychiatric Association (2001) "Practice Guideline for the Treatment of Patients With Borderline Personality Disorder" recommends the use of SSRIs and venlafaxine (at usual antidepressant doses) for treating mood lability, depressed mood, rejection sensitivity, disinhibited anger, impulsivity, and self-damaging behaviors. The positive effects of these antidepressants on impulsive aggression and anger in placebo-controlled studies appeared to be independent of changes in affective symptoms (Coccaro and Kavoussi 1997; Salzman et al. 1995). Lithium augmentation is recommended for patients who have a partial response to an SSRI, whereas a switch to another SSRI is recommended for patients who have no response to an initial SSRI. Atypical antipsychotic agents may be useful but have been less well studied to date (Zanarini et al. 2004). MAOIs also may be effective, particularly in patients with atypical depressive symptoms, but are not recommended as first-line agents because of side effects and the need for dietary restrictions.

■ DISCONTINUATION OF ANTIDEPRESSANTS

Discontinuation of antidepressant medication should be concordant with the guidelines for treatment duration (see "Acute Major Depression" subsection in the preceding section). It is advisable to taper the dose while monitoring for signs and symptoms of relapse. Abrupt discontinuation is also more likely to lead to antidepressant discontinuation symptoms, often referred to as withdrawal symptoms. The occurrence of these symptoms after medication discontinuation does not imply that antidepressants are addictive.

Discontinuation symptoms appear to occur most commonly after discontinuation of short-half-life serotonergic drugs (Coupland et al. 1996), such as fluvoxamine, paroxetine, and venlafaxine.

Patients describe symptoms as flu-like; these symptoms include nausea, diarrhea, insomnia, malaise, muscle aches, anxiety, irritability, dizziness, vertigo, and vivid dreams (Coupland et al. 1996). Often, and for unknown reasons, patients who experience this constellation of symptoms have transient "electric shock" sensations. This unique symptom is diagnostically useful and strongly suggests to the clinician that the patient is in fact experiencing withdrawal because the symptom rarely occurs in other conditions, such as viral infections, or as a side effect of a new medication.

Discontinuation symptoms usually occur within 1–2 days after abrupt discontinuation of a medication and subside within 7–10 days. In some instances, symptoms also may occur during tapering and dose reduction, and they may persist for up to 3 weeks. Restarting treatment with the medication and then tapering more slowly may be necessary, although it is often possible to attenuate withdrawal symptoms produced by short-half-life SSRIs by administering one dose of fluoxetine (which has a longer half-life). In our experience, adding a benzodiazepine for a short period is often helpful.

Abrupt discontinuation of TCAs commonly results in diarrhea, increased sweating, anxiety, and dizziness. These symptoms were previously attributed to cholinergic rebound, but the occurrence of similar symptoms after the discontinuation of many of the newer serotonergic antidepressants suggests that the pathophysiology may be more closely related to changes in serotonin.

■ ANTIDEPRESSANT SWITCHING

Particular care must be exercised when switching from an MAOI to other antidepressant classes. In patients who have completed an MAOI trial without achieving a therapeutic response, treatment with other antidepressants should not be started until 14 days after discontinuation of the original MAOI. Equal care is required when switching from most other antidepressants to an MAOI. An interval equal to five times the half-life of the drug, including active metabolites, is required between stopping treatment with other antidepressant medications and starting MAOI therapy. A 2-week interval is also recommended when switching from phenelzine to tranylcypromine because tranylcypromine is an amphetamine derivative. Theoretically, switching from tranylcypromine, which has a short half-life, to phenelzine should not require as long a waiting period.

Switching between other antidepressants is less problematic. Often clinicians choose to discontinue the first medication before introducing the second one. In most instances, however, a medication-free period is not critical if neither medication is an MAOI. In many instances, it is possible to start administering the new drug while tapering the dose of the first. This overlapping of medications is sometimes helpful to minimize patient discomfort but must be weighed against the risk of increased side effects and drug interactions (Marangell 2001). Considerations to be taken into account when switching antidepressants include half-life and drug interactions.

Switching from one SSRI or SNRI to another can be accomplished by a direct swap of one drug for the next. Although abrupt discontinuation of SSRIs or SNRIs, particularly those with short half-lives, may be associated with discontinuation effects (Rosenbaum et al. 1998), such effects are not seen if another medication is substituted that also inhibits the serotonin reuptake pump. Although both agents will be present until a time equal to five times the half-life of the first medication, this is not usually a problem in practice. Similarly, higher levels of either medication may occur if one or both medications inhibit cytochrome P450 enzymes (e.g., paroxetine or fluoxetine.) This may lead to transient side effects, but it is not usually a safety issue. In most cases, a direct swap is better tolerated than a washing out of the first agent. Although cross-tapering may be useful when medications with different receptor effects are used (e.g., an SSRI and bupropion or mirtazapine), this strategy is not useful when both medications are SSRIs.

■ REFERENCES

American Psychiatric Association: Practice Guideline for the Treatment of Patients With Major Depressive Disorder, 2nd Edition. Washington, DC, American Psychiatric Association, 2000

American Psychiatric Association: Practice Guideline for the Treatment of Patients With Borderline Personality Disorder. Washington, DC, American Psychiatric Association, 2001

Amsterdam J, Berwish NJ: High dose tranylcypromine therapy for refractory depression. Pharmacopsychiatry 22:21–25, 1989

Angst F, Stassen HH, Clayton PJ, et al: Mortality of patients with mood disorders: follow-up over 34–38 years. J Affect Disord 68:167–181, 2002

Anttila AK, Rasanen L, Leinonen EV: Fluvoxamine augmentation increases serum mirtazapine concentrations three- to fourfold. Ann Pharmacother 35:1221–1223, 2001

Arnold LM, Lu Y, Crofford LJ, et al: A double-blind, multicenter trial comparing duloxetine with placebo in the treatment of fibromyalgia patients with or without major depressive disorder. Arthritis Rheum 50:2974–2984, 2004

Boehnert MT, Lovejoy FH: Value of the QRS duration versus the serum drug level in predicting seizures and ventricular arrhythmias after an acute overdose of tricyclic antidepressants. N Engl J Med 313:474–479, 1985

Boyer EW, Shannon M: The serotonin syndrome. N Engl J Med 352:1112–1120, 2005

Bremner JD: A double-blind comparison of Org 3770, amitriptyline, and placebo in major depression. J Clin Psychiatry 56:519–525, 1995

Coccaro EF, Kavoussi RJ: Fluoxetine and impulsive aggressive behavior in personality-disordered subjects. Arch Gen Psychiatry 54:1081–1088, 1997

Coppen A, Mendelwicz J, Kielholz P: Pharmacotherapy of Depressive Disorders: A Consensus Statement. Geneva, World Health Organization, 1986

Coupland NJ, Bell CJ, Potokar JP: Serotonin reuptake inhibitor withdrawal. J Clin Psychopharmacol 16:356–362, 1996

Cymbalta (package insert). Indianapolis, IN, Eli Lilly & Company, 2005

Dalton SO, Johansen C, Mellemkjaer L, et al: Use of selective serotonin reuptake inhibitors and risk of upper gastrointestinal tract bleeding: a population-based cohort study. Arch Intern Med 163:59–64, 2003

Danish University Antidepressant Group: Paroxetine: a selective serotonin reuptake inhibitor showing better tolerance, but weaker antidepressant effect than clomipramine in a controlled multicenter study. J Affect Disord 18:289–299, 1990

de Abajo FJ, Rodriguez LA, Montero D: Association between selective serotonin reuptake inhibitors and upper gastrointestinal bleeding: population based case-control study. BMJ 319:1106–1109, 1999

Demers JC, Malone M: Serotonin syndrome induced by fluvoxamine and mirtazapine. Ann Pharmacother 35:1217–1220, 2001

Depression Guideline Panel: Depression in Primary Care, Vol 2: Treatment of Major Depression (Clinical Practice Guideline No 5; AHCPR Publ No 93-0551). Rockville, MD, U.S. Dept of Health and Human Services, Public Health Service, Agency for Health Care Policy and Research, 1993

Di Rocco A, Brannan T, Prikhojan A, et al: Sertraline induced parkinsonism: a case report and an in-vivo study of the effect of sertraline on dopamine metabolism. J Neural Transm 105:247–251, 1998

Doughty MJ, Lyle WM: Medications used to prevent migraine headaches and their potential ocular adverse effects. Optom Vis Sci 72:879–891, 1995

Fava M, Rankin MA, Alpert JE, et al: An open trial of oral sildenafil in antidepressant-induced sexual dysfunction. Psychother Psychosom 67:328–331, 1998

Fava M, Judge R, Hoog SL, et al: Fluoxetine versus sertraline and paroxetine in major depressive disorder: changes in weight with long-term treatment. J Clin Psychiatry 61:863–867, 2000

Fava M, Thase ME, DeBattista C: A multicenter, placebo-controlled study of modafinil augmentation in partial responders to selective serotonin reuptake inhibitors with persistent fatigue and sleepiness. J Clin Psychiatry 66:85–93, 2005

Frank E, Kupfer DJ, Perel JM, et al: Three-year outcomes for maintenance therapies in recurrent depression. Arch Gen Psychiatry 47:1093–1099, 1990

Gardner DM, Lynd LD: Sumatriptan contraindications and the serotonin syndrome. Ann Pharmacother 32:33–38, 1998

Gardner DM, Shulman KI, Walker SE, et al: The making of a user friendly MAOI diet. J Clin Psychiatry 57:99–104, 1996

Glassman AH, Bigger JT: Cardiovascular effects of therapeutic doses of tricyclic antidepressants: a review. Arch Gen Psychiatry 38:815–820, 1981

Goldberg RJ, Capone RJ, Hunt JD: Cardiac complications following tricyclic antidepressant overdose: issues for monitoring policy. JAMA 254:1772–1775, 1985

Jenike MA: Affective illness in elderly patients, part 2. Psychiatric Times 4:1, 1987

Joffe RT, Singer W: A comparison of triiodothyronine and thyroxine in the potentiation of tricyclic antidepressants. Psychiatry Res 32:241–251, 1990

Joffe RT, Singer W, Levitt AJ, et al: A placebo-controlled comparison of lithium and triiodothyronine augmentation of tricyclic antidepressants in unipolar refractory depression. Arch Gen Psychiatry 50:387–393, 1993

Keller MB: Long-term treatment of recurrent and chronic depression. J Clin Psychiatry 62 (suppl 24):3–5, 2001

Kupfer DJ: Management of recurrent depression. J Clin Psychiatry 54 (suppl 29–33):34–35, 1993

Labbate LA, Pollack MH: Treatment of fluoxetine-induced sexual dysfunction with bupropion: a case report. Ann Clin Psychiatry 6:13–15, 1994

Liebowitz MR, Quitkin FM, Stewart JW, et al: Phenelzine v imipramine in atypical depression: a preliminary report. Arch Gen Psychiatry 41:669–677, 1984

Linazasoro G: Worsening of Parkinson's disease by citalopram. Parkinsonism Relat Disord 6:111–113, 2000

Lingam VR, Lazarus LW, Groves L, et al: Methylphenidate in treating post-stroke depression. J Clin Psychiatry 49:151–153, 1988

Manna V, Bolino F, Di Cicco L: Chronic tension-type headache, mood depression and serotonin: therapeutic effects of fluvoxamine and mianserine. Headache 34:44–49, 1994

Marangell LB: Switching antidepressants for treatment-resistant major depression. J Clin Psychiatry 62 (suppl 18):12–17, 2001

Marangell LB, Johnson CR, Kertz B, et al: Olanzapine in the treatment of apathy in previously depressed participants maintained on SSRIs: an open label, flexible-dose study. J Clin Psychiatry 63:391–395, 2002

Nestler EJ, Barrot M, DiLeone RJ, et al: Neurobiology of depression. Neuron 34:13–25, 2002

Pearlstein TB, Halbreich U, Batzar ED, et al: Psychosocial functioning in women with premenstrual dysphoric disorder before and after treatment with sertraline or placebo. J Clin Psychiatry 61:101–109, 2000

Perry PJ: Pharmacotherapy for major depression with melancholic features: relative efficacy of tricyclic versus selective serotonin reuptake inhibitor antidepressants. J Affect Disord 39:1–6, 1996

Physicians' Desk Reference, 59th Edition. Montvale, NJ, Medical Economics, 2005

Prien RF, Kupfer DJ: Continuation drug therapy for major depression episodes: how long should it be maintained? Am J Psychiatry 143:18–23, 1986

Quitkin F[M], Rifkin A, Klein DF: Monoamine oxidase inhibitors: a review of antidepressant effectiveness. Arch Gen Psychiatry 36:749–760, 1979

Ravaris CL, Robinson DS, Ives JO, et al: Phenelzine and amitriptyline in the treatment of depression: a comparison of present and past studies. Arch Gen Psychiatry 37:1075–1080, 1980

Rosenbaum JF, Fava M, Hoog SL, et al: Selective serotonin reuptake inhibitor discontinuation syndrome: a randomized clinical trial. Biol Psychiatry 44:77–87, 1998

Salzman C, Wolfson AN, Schatzberg A, et al: Effect of fluoxetine on anger in symptomatic volunteers with borderline personality disorder. J Clin Psychopharmacol 15:23–29, 1995

Serzone (package insert). Princeton, NJ, Bristol-Myers Squibb Co, 2002

Smith WT, Glaudin V, Panagides J, et al: Mirtazapine vs. amitriptyline vs. placebo in the treatment of major depressive disorder. Psychopharmacol Bull 26:191–196, 1990

Soloff PH: Psychopharmacology of borderline personality disorder. Psychiatr Clin North Am 23:169–192, 2000

Thase ME: Effects of venlafaxine on blood pressure: a meta-analysis of original data from 3744 depressed patients. J Clin Psychiatry 59:502–508, 1998

Thase ME, Nierenberg AA, Keller MB: Mirtazapine in relapse prevention: a double-blind placebo-controlled study in depressed outpatients. Eur Neuropsychopharmacol 10 (suppl 3):265–266, 2000

Thase ME, Entsuah AR, Rudolph RL: Remission rates during treatment with venlafaxine or selective serotonin reuptake inhibitors. Br J Psychiatry 178:234–241, 2001

U.S. Food and Drug Administration Public Health Advisory: Suicidality in Children and Adolescents Being Treated With Antidepressant Medications, October 15, 2004. Available at: http://www.fda.gov/cder/drug/antidepressants/SSRIPHA200410.htm. Accessed December 7, 2005.

Wehr TA, Goodwin FK: Rapid-cycling in manic depressives induced by tricyclic antidepressants. Arch Gen Psychiatry 36:555–559, 1979

Wikander I, Sundblad C, Andersch B, et al: Citalopram in premenstrual dysphoria: is intermittent treatment during luteal phases more effective than continuous medication throughout the menstrual cycle? J Clin Psychopharmacol 18:390–398, 1998

Yonkers KA, Halbreich U, Freeman E, et al: Symptomatic improvement of premenstrual dysphoric disorder with sertraline treatment: a randomized controlled trial. Sertraline Premenstrual Dysphoric Collaborative Study Group. JAMA 278:983–988, 1997

Zanarini MC, Frankenburg FR, Parachini EA: A preliminary, randomized trial of fluoxetine, olanzapine, and the olanzapine-fluoxetine combination in women with borderline personality disorder. J Clin Psychiatry 65:903–907, 2004

Zisook S: A clinical overview of monoamine oxidase inhibitors. Psychosomatics 26:240–246, 1985

Zyban (package insert). Research Triangle Park, NC, GlaxoSmithKline, 2005

3

ANXIOLYTICS, SEDATIVES, AND HYPNOTICS

Anxiety and insomnia are prevalent symptoms with multiple etiologies. Effective treatments are available, but they vary by diagnosis. In most instances, the best course of action is to treat the underlying disorder rather than reflexively to institute treatment with a nonspecific anxiolytic.

In some cases, anxiolytics serve a transitional purpose. For example, for a patient with acute-onset panic disorder, severe anticipatory anxiety, and a family history of depression, administration of an antidepressant medication that also has antipanic effects may be the optimal treatment, but this will not help the patient for several weeks, during which time there is a risk of progression to agoraphobia. For this patient, starting antidepressant therapy and also attempting to obtain acute symptom relief with a benzodiazepine may be helpful. After 4 weeks, the benzodiazepine dose should be slowly tapered so that the patient's condition is controlled with the antidepressant alone.

In this chapter, we discuss the pharmacology of medications that are classified as anxiolytic, sedative, or hypnotic—primarily the benzodiazepines, buspirone, zolpidem, eszopiclone, and zaleplon. Subsequently, we present diagnosis-specific treatment guidelines (outlined in Table 3–1). The commonly used anxiolytics and hypnotics, together with their usual doses, are shown in Table 3–2. Many antidepressant medications are also effective in the treatment of anxiety disorders. The pharmacology of antidepressants is discussed in Chapter 2; their clinical use in anxiety disorders is addressed in the diagnosis-specific sections later in this chapter.

TABLE 3–1.	Medications of choice for specific anxiety disorders
Diagnosis	**Medication**
Generalized anxiety disorder	Buspirone, benzodiazepines, venlafaxine, SSRIs
Obsessive-compulsive disorder	Clomipramine, SSRIs
Panic disorder	SSRIs, TCAs, MAOIs, benzodiazepines
Performance anxiety	β-Blockers, benzodiazepines
Social phobia	SSRIs, MAOIs, benzodiazepines, buspirone, venlafaxine

Note. SSRIs=selective serotonin reuptake inhibitors; TCAs=tricyclic antidepressants; MAOIs=monoamine oxidase inhibitors.

■ BENZODIAZEPINES

Mechanisms of Action

Benzodiazepines facilitate inhibition by γ-aminobutyric acid (GABA), the major inhibitory neurotransmitter in the brain. The benzodiazepine receptor is a subtype of the $GABA_A$ receptor. Activation of the benzodiazepine receptor facilitates the action of endogenous GABA, which results in the opening of chloride ion channels and a decrease in neuronal excitability. Benzodiazepines act rapidly because ion channels can open and close relatively quickly, in contrast to the slower onset of action that occurs with G protein–linked receptors.

Indications and Efficacy

Benzodiazepines are highly effective anxiolytics and sedatives. They also have muscle relaxant, amnestic, and anticonvulsant properties. Benzodiazepines effectively treat both acute and chronic generalized anxiety and panic disorder. The high-potency benzodiazepines alprazolam and clonazepam have received more attention as antipanic agents, but double-blind studies also have confirmed the efficacy of diazepam and lorazepam in the treatment of panic disorder. Although only a few benzodiazepines are specifically approved by the

TABLE 3–2. Commonly used anxiolytic and hypnotic medications

Drug	Trade name	Single dose (mg)	Usual therapeutic dosage (mg/day)	Approximate dose equivalent (mg)	Methods of administration and supplied forms	Approximate elimination half-life, including metabolites[a]
Benzodiazepines						
Alprazolam	Xanax	0.25–1	1–4	0.5	po: 0.25, 0.5, 1, 2 mg	12 hours
Chlordiazepoxide	Librium	5–25	15–100	10	po: 5, 10, 25 mg; iv, im[b]	1–4 days
Clonazepam	Klonopin	0.5–2	1–4	0.25	po: 0.5, 1, 2 mg	1–2 days
Clorazepate	Tranxene	3.75–22.5	15–60	7.5	po: 3.75, 7.5, 30 mg	2–4 days
Diazepam	Valium	2–10	4–40	5	po: 2, 5, 10 mg; iv, im[b]	2–4 days
Lorazepam	Ativan	0.5–2	1–6	1	po, sl: 0.5, 1, 2 mg; iv, im[b]	12 hours
Oxazepam	Serax	10–30	30–120	15	po: 10, 15, 30 mg	12 hours
Nonbenzodiazepines						
Buspirone	BuSpar	10–30	30–60	NA	po: 5, 10, 15 mg	2–3 hours

Note. po=oral; iv=intravenous; im=intramuscular; sl=sublingual; NA=not applicable.

[a] The clinical duration of action of benzodiazepines does not correlate with the elimination half-life.

[b] Intramuscular lorazepam is well absorbed. We do not recommend intramuscular chlordiazepoxide or diazepam.

Source. Adapted from Teboul and Chouinard 1990.

U.S. Food and Drug Administration for the treatment of insomnia, almost all benzodiazepines may be used for this purpose. Benzodiazepines are most clearly valuable as hypnotics in the hospital setting, where high levels of sensory stimulation, pain, and acute stress may interfere with sleep. The safe, effective, and time-limited use of benzodiazepine hypnotics may, in fact, prevent chronic sleep difficulties (NIMH/NIH Consensus Development Conference Statement 1985). Benzodiazepines are also used to treat akathisia and catatonia and as adjuncts in the treatment of acute mania.

Because alcohol and barbiturates also act, in part, via the $GABA_A$ receptor–mediated chloride ion channel, benzodiazepines show cross-tolerance with these substances. Thus, benzodiazepines are used frequently for treating alcohol or barbiturate withdrawal and detoxification. Alcohol and barbiturates are more dangerous than benzodiazepines because they can act directly at the chloride ion channel at higher doses. In contrast, benzodiazepines have no direct effect on the ion channel; the effects of benzodiazepines are limited by the amount of endogenous GABA.

Selection

At equipotent doses, all benzodiazepines have similar effects. The choice of benzodiazepine is generally based on half-life, rapidity of onset, metabolism, and potency. In patients with moderate to severe hepatic dysfunction, it may be useful to avoid benzodiazepines. All benzodiazepines are metabolized at various levels by the liver, which leads to an increased risk of sedation and confusion in hepatic failure. If it is necessary to prescribe this class of medication, lorazepam and oxazepam are reasonable choices because they are predominantly eliminated by renal excretion.

Risks, Side Effects, and Their Management

Sedation and Impairment of Performance

Benzodiazepine-induced sedation may be considered either a therapeutic action or a side effect. Impairment of performance on sensitive psychomotor tests has been well documented after administration of benzodiazepines. Whether or not sedation is desired, patients must be warned that driving, engaging in dangerous physical activities, and using hazardous machinery should be avoided during the early stages of treatment with benzodiazepines.

Dependence, Withdrawal, and Rebound Effects

Benzodiazepines have a low abuse potential when they are properly prescribed and their use is supervised (American Psychiatric Association 1990). However, physical dependence often occurs when benzodiazepines are taken at higher-than-usual doses or for prolonged periods. If benzodiazepines are discontinued precipitously, withdrawal effects (including hyperpyrexia, seizures, psychosis, and even death) may occur. Signs and symptoms of withdrawal may include tachycardia, increased blood pressure, muscle cramps, anxiety, insomnia, panic attacks, impairment of memory and concentration, perceptual disturbances, and delirium. In addition, withdrawal-related derealization, hallucinations, and other psychotic symptoms have been reported. These withdrawal symptoms may begin as early as the day after discontinuation of the benzodiazepine, and they may continue for weeks to months. Evidence indicates that withdrawal reactions associated with shorter-half-life benzodiazepines peak more rapidly and more intensely.

Most psychoactive medications should be discontinued gradually. For patients who have been taking benzodiazepines for longer than 2–3 months, we suggest that the dose be decreased by approximately 10% per week. Therefore, in the case of a patient receiving alprazolam, 4 mg/day, the dose should be tapered by 0.5 mg/week for 8 weeks.

Memory Impairment

Benzodiazepines are associated with anterograde amnesia, especially when they are administered intravenously and in high doses.

Disinhibition and Dyscontrol

Anecdotal reports suggest that benzodiazepines may occasionally cause paradoxical anger and behavioral disinhibition. A history of hostility, impulsivity, or borderline or antisocial personality disorder is a potential predictor of this reaction. Some caution should be exercised when benzodiazepines are prescribed to patients with a history of poor impulse control and aggression.

Overdose

Benzodiazepines are remarkably safe in overdose. Dangerous effects occur when the overdose includes several sedative drugs, especially alcohol, because of synergistic effects at the chloride ion site and resultant membrane hyperpolarization.

In an emergency setting, the benzodiazepine antagonist flumazenil may be given intravenously to reverse the effects of a potential overdose of a benzodiazepine. Caution in use of flumazenil in a mixed overdose with tricyclic antidepressants (TCAs) is warranted, however. Its use may precipitate TCA-induced arrhythmias and seizures that were suppressed by benzodiazepines.

Drug Interactions

Most sedative drugs, including narcotics and alcohol, potentiate the sedative effects of benzodiazepines. In addition, medications that inhibit hepatic cytochrome P450 (CYP) 3A3/4 increase blood levels and hence side effects of clonazepam, alprazolam, midazolam, and triazolam. Lorazepam, oxazepam, and temazepam are not dependent on hepatic enzymes for metabolism. Therefore, they are not affected by hepatic disease or the inhibition of hepatic enzymes.

Use in Pregnancy

Anxiolytics, like most medications, should be avoided during pregnancy and breast-feeding when possible. There have been concerns that benzodiazepines, when administered during the first trimester of pregnancy, may increase the risk of malformations, particularly cleft palate. Pooled data from cohort studies do not support an increased risk, but data from case-control studies do suggest a risk (Rosenberg et al. 1983). Until further data are available, a high-quality ultrasound should be considered for women who have used benzodiazepines in the first trimester (Dolovich et al. 1998). Some reports have noted that use of benzodiazepines at close proximity to labor may lead to discontinuation symptoms in the neonate, such as hypotonia, apnea, and temperature dysregulation. This risk must be balanced with the risk of the patient's disorder worsening at the time of delivery.

■ BUSPIRONE

Buspirone is a partial agonist at serotonin type 1A (5-HT$_{1A}$) receptors. Unlike benzodiazepines, barbiturates, and alcohol, buspirone does not interact with the GABA receptor or chloride ion channels. Thus, it does not produce sedation, interact with alcohol, impair psychomotor performance, or pose a risk of abuse. There is no cross-tolerance between benzodiazepines and buspirone, so benzodiazepines cannot be abruptly replaced with buspirone. Likewise, buspirone cannot be used to treat alcohol or barbiturate withdrawal and detoxification. Like the antidepressants, buspirone has a relatively slow onset of action.

Indications and Efficacy

Buspirone is effective in the treatment of generalized anxiety. Although the onset of therapeutic action is less rapid, buspirone's efficacy is not statistically different from that of benzodiazepines (Cohn and Wilcox 1986; Goldberg and Finnerty 1979). Despite its success in the treatment of generalized anxiety disorder, buspirone does not appear to be effective against panic disorder (Sheehan et al. 1990), although it might reduce anticipatory anxiety. Buspirone is also used as an augmenting agent in the treatment of obsessive-compulsive disorder (OCD) and depression, and some evidence suggests that buspirone may be an effective treatment for social phobia.

Clinical Use

Buspirone is available for oral administration in a variety of dosage forms. The usual initial dosage is 7.5 mg twice a day, increased after

1 week to 15 mg twice a day. The dose may then be increased as needed to achieve optimal therapeutic response. The usual recommended maximum daily dose is 60 mg, but many patients safely tolerate and benefit from doses up to 90 mg/day. Because buspirone is metabolized by the liver and excreted by the kidneys, it should not be administered to patients with severe hepatic or renal impairment.

Side Effects

The side effects that are more common with buspirone therapy than with benzodiazepine therapy are nausea, headache, nervousness, insomnia, dizziness, and light-headedness. Restlessness also has been reported.

Overdose

No fatal outcomes of buspirone overdose have been reported. However, overdose of buspirone with other drugs may result in more serious outcomes.

Drug Interactions

Buspirone is metabolized by CYP 3A3/4. Therefore, the initial dose should be lower in patients who are also taking medications known to inhibit these enzymes, such as nefazodone.

Buspirone should not be administered in combination with a monoamine oxidase inhibitor (MAOI).

■ ZOLPIDEM AND ZALEPLON

Zolpidem and zaleplon are hypnotics that act at the omega-1 receptor of the central $GABA_A$ receptor complex. This selectivity is hypothesized to be associated with a lower risk of dependence. Unlike benzodiazepines, zolpidem and zaleplon do not appear to have significant anxiolytic, muscle relaxant, or anticonvulsant properties. However, amnestic effects may occur.

Indications and Efficacy

Zolpidem is a short-acting hypnotic with established efficacy in inducing and maintaining sleep. Because of the short half-life of this drug, most patients taking zolpidem report minimal daytime sedation.

Zaleplon is an ultra-short-acting hypnotic and can therefore be administered in the middle of the night; minimal residual sedative effects occur after 4 hours.

Trials of different modified-release formulations of zaleplon, zolpidem, and a similar selective $GABA_A$ hypnotic, indiplon, are ongoing. These versions may help improve the sleep of those patients who have sleep maintenance insomnia or early-morning awakening.

Clinical Use

Both zolpidem and zaleplon are available in 5- and 10-mg tablets for oral administration. The maximum recommended dose for adults is 10 mg/day and 20 mg/day, respectively, administered at night. The initial dose for elderly persons should not exceed 5 mg. Caution is advised in patients with hepatic dysfunction. In general, hypnotics should be limited to short-term use, with reevaluation for more extended therapy (see below under "Treatment of Specific Conditions").

Side Effects

In general, side effects of zolpidem and zaleplon are similar to those of short-acting benzodiazepines. These agents should not be considered free of abuse potential.

Overdose

Both zolpidem and zaleplon appear to be nonfatal in overdose. However, overdoses in combination with other central nervous system (CNS) depressant agents pose a greater risk. Recommended treatment consists of general symptomatic and supportive measures, including gastric lavage. Use of flumazenil may be helpful.

Drug Interactions

Research on drug interactions with zolpidem and zaleplon is limited, but any drug with CNS depressant effects could potentially enhance the CNS depressant effects of zolpidem and zaleplon through pharmacodynamic interactions. In addition, zolpidem is primarily metabolized by CYP 3A3/4, and zaleplon is partially metabolized by CYP 3A3/4. Thus, inhibitors of these enzymes may increase blood levels and the toxicity of zolpidem.

■ RAMELTEON

Ramelteon is a hypnotic with melatonin receptor agonist activity targeting melatonin MT_1 and MT_2 receptors. It has not been proven to induce dependence. As with zolpidem and zaleplon, no known anxiolytic properties have been elicited. No appreciable activity on serotonin, dopamine, GABA, or acetylcholine is present with the parent compound, but in vitro studies report that its primary metabolite M-II has weak $5\text{-}HT_{2B}$ receptor agonist activity.

Indications and Efficacy

Ramelteon is indicated for the treatment of insomnia, specifically, to improve sleep latency. Because its half-life is 1–2.6 hours, this medication is not thought to be associated with daytime sedation.

Clinical Use

Ramelteon is available in 8-mg tablets for oral administration. The current maximum dosage is 8 mg administered at night; however, during trials, up to 16 mg was studied. Ramelteon should be used with caution in elderly patients because plasma levels were twice those in healthy adults in clinical trials. Ramelteon should not be used by patients with severe hepatic impairment. This medication has been evaluated in moderate sleep apnea and chronic obstructive pulmonary disease and appeared to be safe to administer in this population. Ramelteon was not studied in subjects with severe sleep apnea or severe chronic obstructive pulmonary disease and is not recommended for use in these patients.

Side Effects

The most common side effects (>2% incidence difference from placebo) were somnolence, dizziness, and fatigue.

Ramelteon has been associated with decreased testosterone levels and increased prolactin levels. No studies have been performed in children or adolescents with this medication. Trials of ramelteon have not indicated high abuse potential.

Overdose

Ramelteon in doses up to 160 mg has been studied and appears to be nonfatal in overdose. Supportive measures are recommended if overdose occurs. Gastric lavage also should be considered.

Drug Interactions

Ramelteon is metabolized by the hepatic system; CYP 1A2 is the major isoenzyme involved. Caution is recommended with other inhibitory agents such as fluvoxamine. Ramelteon is metabolized to a lesser extent through CYP 3A4 and 2C9, and additional caution is necessary with drugs affecting these portions of the cytochrome P450 system.

■ ESZOPICLONE

Eszopiclone is an additional hypnotic thought to act on GABA receptor complexes close to benzodiazepine receptors. No anxiolytic effect has been documented in the literature on this medication.

Indications and Efficacy

Eszopiclone is short acting, with a half-life of approximately 6 hours. Its efficacy is established in inducing and maintaining sleep. Its duration of action is estimated to be approximately 8 hours, similar to zolpidem.

Clinical Use

Eszopiclone is available in 1-, 2-, and 3-mg tablets for oral administration. The maximum recommended dose is 3 mg/night. In the elderly, this dose is reduced to maximum of 2 mg. No evidence of tolerance or dependence has been reported, but long-term use should be approached with caution. In addition, eszopiclone should be used cautiously in substance abuse patients because trials have shown euphoric effects at high doses.

Side Effects

Eszopiclone has side effects similar to those of other short-acting benzodiazepines. Dizziness, headache, and unpleasant taste were the most commonly reported side effects in patients taking eszopiclone in clinical trials.

Overdose

Limited information on overdose with eszopiclone is available at this time. No fatalities have been reported with up to 36 mg being taken in overdose. Overdose symptoms include impairment in consciousness, including somnolence or coma. Treatment is symptomatic driven and supportive. Flumazenil may be beneficial.

Drug Interactions

Eszopiclone is metabolized in the liver by CYP 3A4. Eszopiclone should not be used in patients with severe hepatic impairment. Dose adjustment and caution are recommended in patients taking enzyme inhibitors such as ketoconazole, ciprofloxacin, erythromycin, isoniazid, and nefazodone. Other sedative-hypnotics are not recommended with administration of this medication.

■ TREATMENT OF SPECIFIC CONDITIONS

Generalized Anxiety Disorder

Generalized anxiety disorder can be treated with benzodiazepines, buspirone, and certain antidepressants (e.g., venlafaxine, paroxetine, escitalopram). These agents are compared in Table 3–3.

Benzodiazepines have the advantage of being rapidly effective but the obvious disadvantages of abuse potential and sedation. Although benzodiazepines are indicated for relatively short-term use only (i.e., 1–2 months), they are generally safe and effective when used for long periods. Whereas tolerance to sedation often develops, the same is not true of the anxiolytic effects of these agents. All benzodiazepines indicated for the treatment of anxiety are equally efficacious. The choice of a specific agent usually depends on the pharmacokinetics and pharmacodynamics of the drug. Some patients respond to extremely low dosages, such as 0.125 mg of alprazolam twice a day, although mean doses are typically higher. When benzodiazepines are used to treat anxiety, the clinician should start with alprazolam, 0.25 mg two or three times a day or an equivalent dosage of another benzodiazepine (Table 3–2), and then titrate the dose to achieve maximal anxiolytic effect and minimal sedation. Benzodiazepines should be avoided in patients with a history of recent and/or significant substance abuse, and all patients should be advised to take the first dose at home in a situation that would not be dangerous in the event of greater-than-expected sedation.

Unlike benzodiazepines, buspirone is not associated with sedative or abuse problems, but some clinicians have observed that buspirone's anxiolytic properties do not appear to be as potent as those of benzodiazepines, particularly in patients who have previously received a benzodiazepine. Because buspirone is not sedating and has no psychomotor effects, it has a distinct advantage over benzodiazepines when optimal alertness and motor performance are necessary. Response to buspirone occurs in approximately 2–4 weeks. Buspirone does not show cross-tolerance with benzodiazepines and other sedative or hypnotic drugs such as alcohol, barbiturates, and chloral hydrate. Therefore, buspirone does not suppress benzodiazepine withdrawal symptoms. In anxious patients who are taking a benzodiazepine and who require a switch to buspirone, the benzodiazepine must be tapered gradually to avoid withdrawal symptoms, despite the fact that the patient is receiving buspirone.

Generalized anxiety disorder also responds to antidepressant treatment; response occurs in approximately 2–3 weeks, but maxi-

TABLE 3–3. Comparison of benzodiazepines, buspirone, and antidepressants for the treatment of anxiety

Characteristic	Benzodiazepines	Buspirone	Antidepressants[a]
Therapeutic effect of single dose	Yes	No	No
Time to full therapeutic action	Days	Weeks	Weeks
Sedation	Yes	No	Unlikely
Dependence liability	Yes	No	No
Impairs performance	Yes	No	No
Suppresses sedative withdrawal symptoms	Yes	No	No
Once-daily dosing	No	No	Yes
Treats comorbid depression	No	No	Yes
Side effects	Sedation, memory impairment	Dizziness	Gastrointestinal effects, sexual dysfunction

[a]See text for details.

mal response may take months. Venlafaxine, escitalopram, and paroxetine have received U.S. Food and Drug Administration approval for this indication, although it is likely that the other selective serotonin reuptake inhibitors (SSRIs) are effective as well.

The duration of pharmacotherapy for generalized anxiety disorder is controversial. Psychotherapy is recommended for most patients with this disorder, and it may facilitate the tapering of doses of medication. However, generalized anxiety is often a chronic condition, and some patients require long-term pharmacotherapy. As in other anxiety disorders, the need for ongoing treatment should be reassessed every 6–12 months.

Panic Disorder

Benzodiazepines, TCAs, MAOIs, and SSRIs are all effective in the treatment of panic disorder. Among the benzodiazepines, the higher-potency agents alprazolam and clonazepam are preferred because they are well tolerated at the higher doses often required to treat panic disorder. Clonazepam has the advantage of a longer elimination half-life, which results in more stable plasma drug levels and allows twice-daily dosing. The shorter half-life of alprazolam, conversely, makes that drug better suited for acute dose titration. For the treatment of panic disorder, clonazepam therapy is started at 0.5 mg twice a day, and the dose is increased to a total of 1–2 mg/day in two divided doses. Higher dose levels may be necessary for complete relief of symptoms. The starting dosage of alprazolam is usually 0.25 or 0.5 mg three times a day.

Because long-term exposure to high-dose benzodiazepines may place some patients at risk for physical and psychological dependence, we recommend the use of antidepressants for the treatment of panic disorder. For most patients, SSRIs should be considered first-line agents. The choice should be based on the factors discussed in Chapter 2. MAOIs are usually reserved for patients whose symptoms have not responded to SSRIs and TCAs. A major caveat is that patients with panic disorder initially may be highly sensitive to the stimulant effect of small doses of antidepressants. For highly anxious patients with panic disorder, treatment may be initiated with clonazepam or alprazolam and an antidepressant at a low dose, which is then increased slowly. The rapid onset of action of the benzodiazepine is helpful to the patient until the antidepressant becomes effective. When panic symptoms have been absent for several weeks, the benzodiazepine dose is slowly tapered. In patients with marked residual anticipatory anxiety, longer-term use of a benzodiazepine or buspirone should be considered as an adjunct to treatment with the antidepressant. Although some patients respond to lower doses, standard or high-standard antidepressant doses generally are used for the treatment of panic disorder.

Unfortunately, no guidelines exist for the duration of pharmacotherapy. We recommend attempting to discontinue medication gradually every 6–12 months if the patient has been relatively symptom-free. However, many patients require longer-term pharmacotherapy.

Social Phobia

Social phobia responds to a variety of medications, including SSRIs, MAOIs, benzodiazepines, and buspirone. TCAs, although highly effective in the treatment of panic disorder, appear to be ineffective for most patients with social phobia. Similarly, β-blockers, although effective against performance anxiety, are typically not effective in treating generalized social phobia. Dosages for the treatment of social phobia are similar to dosages of these medications for the treatment of other disorders.

Performance Anxiety

Several studies have reported the efficacy of β-blockers in the treatment of performance anxiety. Taken within 2 hours of a stressful event (e.g., an examination, a speech, or a concert), propranolol, 20–80 mg, may improve performance. A trial dose of 40 mg of propranolol should be administered before the performance situation in which the patient anticipates anxiety. This initial dose should not be taken in a high-risk or critical situation in which any unexpected side effect could have serious consequences. Subsequently, doses of propranolol should be administered approximately 2 hours before the situation in which disabling performance anxiety is expected. The dose may be increased gradually in 20-mg increments during successive performances until adequate relief of performance distress is achieved.

Obsessive-Compulsive Disorder

The TCA clomipramine and the SSRIs provide the foundation of the pharmacological treatment for OCD. Although pharmacotherapy is effective against many other Axis I disorders, most patients with OCD experience only a 35%–60% improvement in symptoms. In addition, medication responses may not be apparent until treatment has been administered for 10 weeks, and some patients will require higher doses than are typically used to treat depression. As in the treatment of depression, SSRIs tend to be better tolerated than TCAs (clomipramine is the only effective TCA for OCD).

Several augmentation strategies have been suggested. None has been associated with uniformly positive results in controlled trials, but possible effectiveness has been noted in selected patients. Augmentation strategies for OCD include the use of lithium, antipsychotics, clonazepam, or buspirone.

As in other anxiety disorders, relatively few data are available on longer-term treatment of OCD. OCD is often a lifelong disorder with a waxing and waning course, for which many patients require prolonged pharmacotherapy.

Insomnia

Although benzodiazepines, zolpidem, zaleplon, and eszopiclone are the mainstay of pharmacotherapy for insomnia, other sedating drugs, such as trazodone, diphenhydramine, or chloral hydrate, also may be used. Insomnia should first be addressed diagnostically, and in most cases, nonpharmacological interventions should be attempted before treatment with a hypnotic is instituted. Hypnotic agents should be administered in the lowest effective dose. Medications commonly prescribed for insomnia, along with their recommended doses, times of onset, and half-lives, are shown in Table 3–4. General principles for using medications to treat insomnia are outlined in Table 3–5.

Alcohol Withdrawal

A relatively simple procedure for treating alcohol withdrawal is the benzodiazepine loading-dose technique. This technique takes advantage of the long half-lives of benzodiazepines such as diazepam and chlordiazepoxide. For example, patients receive 100-mg doses of chlordiazepoxide every hour until no signs or symptoms of alcohol withdrawal are observed. This state is usually accompanied by mild to moderate sedation. Thereafter, no further doses of the benzodiazepine are administered. Healthy patients should receive at least 300 mg of chlordiazepoxide in the initial loading-dose regimen. This technique has advantages over repeat dosing with benzodiazepines; with the latter method, the accumulation of benzodiazepines may lead to prolonged sedation and the development of benzodiazepine dependence in a population at high risk for chemical dependence. For patients with hepatic disease, the use of lorazepam or oxazepam should be considered.

Substance Abuse and Anxiety

For those with a history of substance abuse or intolerance to benzodiazepines and the elderly, caution must be used in controlling anxiety. In these cases, benzodiazepines may exacerbate other conditions. Preliminary reports suggest that antipsychotics such as quetiapine may alleviate symptoms of anxiety. Other strategies include use of antihistamines such as hydroxyzine and diphenhydramine.

Agitation and Aggression

Whereas benzodiazepines are frequently used for the treatment of acute agitation in medical settings, data are inconsistent on the effects of benzodiazepines on aggression. The overarching principle

TABLE 3–4. Medications commonly prescribed for insomnia

Medication	Trade name	Usual therapeutic dosage (mg/day)		Time until onset of action (minutes)	Half-life, including metabolites (hours)
		Adult	Geriatric		
Clonazepam[a]	Klonopin	0.5–2	0.25–1	20–60	19–60
Clorazepate	Tranxene	3.75–15	3.75–7.5	30–60	48–96
Estazolam	ProSom	1–2	0.5–1	15–30	8–24
Eszopiclone	Lunesta	3	2	60	6–9
Flurazepam	Dalmane	30	15	30–60	100
Lorazepam[a]	Ativan	1–4	0.25–1	30–60	8–24
Oxazepam	Serax	15–30	10–15	30–60	2.8–5.7
Quazepam	Doral	7.5–15	7.5	20–45	39–120
Temazepam	Restoril	15–30	7.5–15	45–60	3–25
Triazolam	Halcion	0.125–0.25	0.125	15–30	1.5–5
Chloral hydrate[b]	(none)	500–2,000	500–2,000	30–60	4–8
Trazodone[a,b]	Desyrel	50–150	25–100	30–60	5–9
Zolpidem[b]	Ambien	5–10	5	30	1.5–4.5
Zaleplon[b]	Sonata	5–10	5	30	1.0

[a]Use as a hypnotic is not an indication approved by the U.S. Food and Drug Administration.
[b]Not a benzodiazepine.

Source.   Adapted from Kupfer and Reynolds 1997, with additional information from Physicians' Desk Reference 2005.

TABLE 3–5.   **Guidelines for pharmacotherapy for insomnia**

Use the lowest effective dose.
Use agents with short or intermediate half-lives to avoid daytime sedation.
Use intermittent dosing (two to four times a week).
Use for no more than 3–4 weeks.
Discontinue medication gradually.
Be alert for rebound insomnia.

Source.   Adapted from Kupfer and Reynolds 1997.

to keep in mind when establishing a treatment plan for a patient with agitation or aggression is that diagnosis comes before treatment. After appropriate assessment of possible etiologies of these behaviors, treatment is focused on the occurrence of comorbid neuropsychiatric conditions (depression, psychosis, insomnia, anxiety, delirium). The sedative properties of benzodiazepines are helpful in the management of acute agitation or aggression, but these agents should not be used chronically. Benzodiazepines can produce amnesia, and preexisting memory dysfunction can be exacerbated by the use of benzodiazepines. Brain-injured patients also may experience increased problems with coordination and balance with benzodiazepine use.

For the treatment of acute aggression or agitation, lorazepam, 1–2 mg, may be administered orally or intramuscularly every hour until sedation is achieved (Silver and Yudofsky 1994). Intravenous lorazepam is also effective, although the onset of action is similar to that for intramuscular administration. Caution must be taken with intravenous administration, and the agent should be injected in doses less than 1 mg/minute to avoid laryngospasm. Gradual tapering of the lorazepam dose may be attempted when the patient's aggressive or agitated behavior has been in control for 48 hours. If aggressive behavior recurs, medications for the treatment of chronic aggression (e.g., anticonvulsants, propranolol) may be given. If necessary, lorazepam may be administered in combination with an antipsychotic medication (e.g., risperidone, 1–2 mg). Antipsychotic medications (see Chapter 4) are also used for acute agitation, especially in psychotic patients.

■ REFERENCES

American Psychiatric Association: Benzodiazepine Dependence, Toxicity, and Abuse: A Task Force Report of the American Psychiatric Association. Washington, DC, American Psychiatric Association, 1990

Cohn JB, Wilcox CS: Low-sedation potential of buspirone compared with alprazolam and lorazepam in the treatment of anxious patients: a double-blind study. J Clin Psychiatry 47:409–412, 1986

Dolovich LR, Addis A, Vaillancourt JM, et al: Benzodiazepine use in pregnancy and major malformations or oral cleft: meta-analysis of cohort and case-control studies. BMJ 317:839–843, 1998

Goldberg HL, Finnerty RJ: The comparative efficacy of buspirone and diazepam in the treatment of anxiety. Am J Psychiatry 136:1184–1187, 1979

Kupfer DJ, Reynolds CF III: Management of insomnia. N Engl J Med 336:341–346, 1997

NIMH/NIH Consensus Development Conference Statement: Mood disorders: pharmacologic prevention of recurrences. Consensus Development Panel. Am J Psychiatry 142:469–476, 1985

Physicians' Desk Reference, 59th Edition. Montvale, NJ, Medical Economics, 2005

Rosenberg L, Mitchell AA, Parsells JL, et al: Lack of relation of oral clefts to diazepam use during pregnancy. N Engl J Med 309:1282–1285, 1983

Sheehan DV, Raj AB, Sheehan KH, et al: Is buspirone effective for panic disorder? J Clin Psychopharmacol 10:3–11, 1990

Silver JM, Yudofsky SC: Aggressive disorders, in Neuropsychiatry of Traumatic Brain Injury. Edited by Silver JM, Yudofsky SC, Hales RE. Washington, DC, American Psychiatric Press, 1994, pp 313–353

Teboul E, Chouinard G: A guide to benzodiazepine selection, part 1: pharmacological aspects. Can J Psychiatry 35:700–710, 1990

4

ANTIPSYCHOTICS

Antipsychotic medications, previously referred to as major tranquilizers or neuroleptics, are effective for the treatment of a variety of psychotic symptoms—such as hallucinations, delusions, and thought disorders—regardless of etiology. The term *major tranquilizer* is a misnomer because sedation is generally a side effect, and not the principal treatment effect. Similarly, the term *neuroleptic* is based on the neurological side effects characteristic of older antipsychotic drugs, such as catalepsy in animals and extrapyramidal side effects (EPS) in humans.

Antipsychotic drugs can be classified in several ways. One classification is based on chemical structure; for example, phenothiazines and butyrophenones make up two chemical classes. We use the term *conventional* to signify older or first-generation antipsychotic drugs—to differentiate them from newer, atypical or second-generation antipsychotics. All conventional antipsychotics are equally effective when given in equivalent doses (Table 4–1). Among the conventional antipsychotics, we commonly distinguish between high- and low-potency agents, because the level of potency predicts side effects. Although the term *atypical antipsychotic* lacks a single consistent definition, it generally implies fewer EPS and superior efficacy, particularly for the negative symptoms of schizophrenia. Atypical antipsychotics are also less likely to produce hyperprolactinemia. Atypical antipsychotics include clozapine, risperidone, olanzapine, quetiapine, ziprasidone, and aripiprazole.

The efficacy and favorable neurological side-effect profiles of atypical antipsychotics have led to the recommendation for their uniform use as first-line agents—with the exception of clozapine,

TABLE 4–1. Commonly used antipsychotic drugs

Drug	Trade name	Usual daily dose (mg)	Methods and forms of administration	Available oral doses (mg)	Approximate oral dose equivalents (mg)
Atypical antipsychotics					
Aripiprazole	Abilify	15–30	po, L	5, 10, 15, 20, 30; 1 mg/mL	4
Clozapine	Clozaril	250–500	po, ODT	25, 100	100
Olanzapine	Zyprexa	10–20	po, ODT; im	2.5, 5, 7.5, 10, 15, 20	4
Quetiapine	Seroquel	300–600	po	25, 100, 200, 300	125
Risperidone	Risperdal	4–6	po, L, ODT, D	0.25, 0.5, 1, 2, 3, 4; 1 mg/mL	1
Ziprasidone	Geodon	80–160	po, im	20, 40, 60, 80	40
Conventional antipsychotics					
Butyrophenones					
Droperidol	Inapsine	2.5–10	im	2.5 mg/ml	—
Haloperidol	Haldol	5–15	po, im, D	0.5, 1, 2, 5, 10, 20	2
Dibenzoxazepines					
Loxapine	Loxitane	45–90	po	5, 10, 25, 50	10
Dihydroindolones					
Molindone	Moban	30–60	po	5, 10, 25, 50	15

TABLE 4–1. Commonly used antipsychotic drugs *(continued)*

Drug	Trade name	Usual daily dose (mg)	Methods and forms of administration	Available oral doses (mg)	Approximate oral dose equivalents (mg)
Phenothiazines					
Aliphatics					
Chlorpromazine	Thorazine	300–600	po, L, im	10, 25, 50, 100, 200; 100 mg/mL	100
Piperazines					
Fluphenazine	Prolixin	5–15	po, L, im, D	1, 2.5, 5, 10	2
Perphenazine	Trilafon, Etrafon	32–64	po, L	2, 4, 8, 16; 16 mg/mL	10
Trifluoperazine	Stelazine	5–30	po	1, 2, 5, 10	5
Piperidines					
Mesoridazine	Serentil	150–300	po	10, 25, 50, 100	50
Thioridazine	Mellaril	300–600	po, im	10, 15, 25, 50, 100	100
Diphenylbutylpiperidine					
Pimozide	Orap	2–6	po	1, 2	2
Thioxanthenes					
Thiothixene	Navane	5–30	po, L	1, 2, 5, 10, 20; 5 mg/mL	4

Note. po=oral tablets or capsules; L=liquid; ODT=oral disintegrating tablets; im=intramuscular injections; D=decanoate.
Source. Equivalent doses from Fuller and Sajatovic 2004.

whose use is restricted because of the risk of agranulocytosis (Lieberman 1996). This chapter begins with a discussion of the properties common to most antipsychotic medications, continues with specific comments on each atypical antipsychotic, and concludes with treatment principles for schizophrenia. The use of antipsychotic medications to treat other disorders is addressed elsewhere in this book.

■ MECHANISMS OF ACTION

Underactivity of dopamine in mesocortical pathways, specifically those projecting to the frontal lobes, may account for the negative symptoms of schizophrenia (e.g., anergia, apathy, lack of spontaneity) (Davis et al. 1991; Goff and Evins 1998). In addition, this underactivity in the frontal lobes may serve to disinhibit mesolimbic dopamine activity via a corticolimbic feedback loop. Overactivity of mesolimbic dopamine is the result, which manifests as the positive symptoms of schizophrenia (e.g., hallucinations, delusions).

Antipsychotic medications antagonize dopamine, which is believed to contribute to the antipsychotic effect of these medications. The atypical antipsychotics have other physiological properties as well, some of which appear to relate to antagonism of the serotonin type 2 (5-HT_2) receptor, which may modify dopamine activity in a regionally specific manner. Dual 5-HT_2 receptor–dopamine type 2 (D_2) receptor antagonism is believed to account, at least in part, for the superior efficacy and more favorable side-effect profile of atypical antipsychotics.

■ INDICATIONS AND EFFICACY

The most common indications for antipsychotic drugs are the treatment of acute psychosis and the maintenance of remission of psychotic symptoms in patients with schizophrenia. More recently, the atypical antipsychotics have become part of the standard repertoire for the treatment of bipolar disorder, as discussed in Chapter 5. Antipsychotic drugs also ameliorate psychotic symptoms associated with drug intoxications, delusional disorders, and nonspecific agitation, although the data supporting their use in these conditions are limited. In addition, low doses of antipsychotics may be effective in some patients with borderline or schizotypal personality disorders, particularly when psychotic ideation is targeted (Oldham 2005). In patients with severe obsessive-compulsive disorder, antipsychotics have been used to augment treatment with antiobsessional agents. Antipsychotics and other drugs with dopamine receptor–blocking action (e.g., metoclopramide) are also used for their antiemetic effect. Lastly, Gilles de la Tourette's syndrome may be controlled with antipsychotic agents; haloperidol and pimozide are the most frequently used drugs for this disorder.

■ CLINICAL USE

As with antidepressant therapy, reversal of psychosis is often gradual and may occur over several weeks to several months. Guidelines for the acute use of antipsychotic drugs are summarized in Table 4–2; usual dosages for each of the commonly used antipsychotic drugs are summarized in Table 4–1.

■ MEDICATION SELECTION

The choice of antipsychotic medication is often determined, in large part, by anticipated side effects. In most circumstances, atypical antipsychotics (except for clozapine) are best tolerated and are preferred as first-line agents. Clozapine is generally reserved for patients with refractory illness because of the risk of agranulocytosis.

■ RISKS, SIDE EFFECTS, AND THEIR MANAGEMENT

Many side effects of antipsychotic drugs can be understood in terms of the drugs' receptor-blocking properties. When antipsychotics reduce dopamine activity in the nigrostriatal pathway (via dopamine

TABLE 4–2.	Guidelines for the acute use of antipsychotic drugs

1. Before initiating treatment, obtain a medical history and a psychiatric history. Baseline laboratory studies are also indicated if they have not already been completed as part of the initial evaluation of the patient. An evaluation for the presence of any abnormal movements is also advisable. An electrocardiogram should be considered for patients with a history of cardiac problems.

2. After discussion with the patient and family about the risks and benefits of treatment, select the appropriate antipsychotic agent on the basis of the patient's physical status, the side-effect profile of the drug, and the patient's previous responses to medication, if known.

3. Educate the patient and family about the risks of developing metabolic syndrome, diabetes, obesity, dyslipidemia, and tardive dyskinesia. Document this discussion in the patient's chart.

4. Initiate treatment with antipsychotic medications at low to moderate doses, depending on the patient's history and clinical presentation. Titrate as tolerated to the target dose (Table 4–1).

5. In patients with acute agitation, a sedative such as lorazepam (2 mg) may be effective.

6. If possible, give all antipsychotic medication at bedtime to increase compliance and minimize daytime side effects.

7. If the patient has been compliant with treatment, side effects are minimal, and there is no or minimal response to treatment, increase the dose gradually (e.g., every 2–4 weeks). Full response may be delayed for 6 months or longer.

8. If there is still no response, the patient is taking an adequate dose, and the patient is adherent with treatment, consider another antipsychotic.

Source.   Lehman et al. 2004.

receptor blockade), extrapyramidal signs and symptoms similar to those of Parkinson's disease result. Another locus of dopamine receptors is in the pituitary and hypothalamus (the tuberoinfundibular system), where dopamine is synonymous with prolactin-inhibiting factor. Blockade of dopamine in this system results in hyper-prolactinemia. Similarly, antagonism of acetylcholine receptors produces symptoms such as dry mouth, blurred vision, and constipation. Antagonism of α_1-adrenergic receptors results in hypotension, and antagonism of histamine receptors is associated with sedation.

Extrapyramidal Side Effects

EPS include acute dystonic reactions, parkinsonian syndrome, akathisia, tardive dyskinesia, and neuroleptic malignant syndrome. Although high-potency conventional antipsychotics are more likely than low-potency conventional antipsychotics to cause EPS, all first-generation antipsychotic drugs are equally likely to cause tardive dyskinesia. The atypical antipsychotics cause substantially fewer EPS, which is one reason that they are recommended as first-line agents.

Acute Dystonic Reactions

Acute dystonic reactions occur within hours or days of initiation of treatment with a high-potency conventional antipsychotic medication. The uncontrollable tightening of muscles typically involves spasms of the neck, back (opisthotonos), tongue, or muscles that control lateral eye movement (oculogyric crisis). Laryngeal involvement may compromise the airway and result in ventilatory difficulties (stridor). Intravenous or intramuscular administration of anticholinergic medication is a rapid and effective treatment for acute dystonia. The drugs and dosages used to treat dystonic reactions are listed in Table 4–3. The effects of the anticholinergic drug given to reverse the dystonia wear off after several hours. Because antipsychotic drugs have long half-lives and durations of action, additional oral anticholinergic drugs should be prescribed for several days after an acute dystonic reaction, or longer if treatment with the antipsychotic drug is continued unchanged. Amantadine, 100 mg twice a day, should be considered for treatment of EPS in elderly patients who are highly sensitive to anticholinergic activity.

TABLE 4–3. Drugs commonly used to treat acute extrapyramidal side effects

Drug	Drug type	Usual dosage	Indications
Amantadine	Dopaminergic agent	100 mg po bid	Parkinsonian syndrome
Benztropine	Anticholinergic agent	1–2 mg po bid 2 mg iv[a]	Dystonia, parkinsonian syndrome Acute dystonia
Diphenhydramine	Anticholinergic agent	25–50 mg po tid 25 mg im or iv[a]	Dystonia, parkinsonian syndrome Acute dystonia
Propranolol	β-Blocker	20 mg po tid 1 mg iv	Akathisia
Trihexyphenidyl	Anticholinergic agent	5–10 mg po bid	Dystonia, parkinsonian syndrome

Note. po=oral tablets or capsules; bid=twice daily; iv=intravenous; tid=three times a day; im=intramuscular injections.
[a]Follow with oral medication.

Parkinsonian Syndrome

Parkinsonian syndrome (or pseudoparkinsonism) has many of the features of classic idiopathic Parkinson's disease: diminished range of facial expression (masked facies), cogwheel rigidity, slowed movements (bradykinesia), drooling, small handwriting (micrographia), and pill-rolling tremor. As in Parkinson's disease, the pathophysiology involves the presence of disproportionately less dopamine than acetylcholine in the basal ganglia. The onset of this side effect is gradual, and the side effect may not appear for weeks after antipsychotics have been administered. The most common treatments for idiopathic Parkinson's disease restore the dopamine–acetylcholine balance by increasing dopamine availability. Because dopamine antagonism is putatively involved in the therapeutic effects of antipsychotics, treatment of parkinsonism most often involves decreasing the level of acetylcholine (although amantadine, a dopaminergic drug, often effectively attenuates parkinsonian side effects without exacerbating the underlying psychotic illness). Drugs used in the treatment of the parkinsonian side effects of antipsychotic agents are listed in Table 4–3.

Akathisia

Akathisia is an extrapyramidal disorder consisting of a subjective feeling of restlessness in the lower extremities, often manifested as an inability to sit still. It is a common reaction that most often occurs shortly after initiation of treatment with a conventional antipsychotic medication or aripiprazole. Treatment options for akathisia include switching from a conventional antipsychotic to an atypical antipsychotic, adding a β-adrenergic-blocking drug (particularly propranolol in doses up to 120 mg/day), lowering the dose of aripiprazole, or switching from aripiprazole to a different atypical antipsychotic.

Tardive Disorders

Tardive dyskinesia is a disorder characterized by involuntary choreoathetoid movements of the face, trunk, or extremities. The syndrome is usually associated with prolonged exposure to dopamine receptor–blocking agents—most frequently, antipsychotic drugs. The American Psychiatric Association Task Force on Tardive Dyskinesia estimated a cumulative incidence of 5% per year of exposure among young adults and a prevalence of 30% after 1 year of treatment with conventional antipsychotics among elderly patients (American Psychiatric Association 1992). Clozapine seems to carry little or no risk of inducing tardive dyskinesia. The incidence of tardive dyskinesia associated with other atypical antipsychotics is higher than that associated with clozapine and lower than that associated with conventional antipsychotics (Correll et al. 2004; Jeste et al. 1999; Tollefson et al. 1997). Elderly patients taking antipsychotics are at increased risk for tardive dyskinesia.

If discontinuation of the antipsychotic drug is clinically possible, gradual improvement of tardive dyskinesia may occur, although involuntary movements often worsen initially with tapering of the antipsychotic dose, a phenomenon referred to as *withdrawal-emergent dyskinesia* (Glazer et al. 1984). Withdrawal-emergent dyskinesia also may appear when a conventional antipsychotic is replaced with an atypical antipsychotic. Withdrawal-emergent dyskinesia typically resolves within 6 weeks.

There is no definitive treatment for tardive dyskinesia. In several small studies, α-tocopherol (vitamin E) was shown to be of some benefit. The typical dose of vitamin E is 1,600 IU/day. Clozapine may be useful for certain patients with TD who need an antipsychotic alternative. In a clinical study by Lieberman et al. (1991), 30 patients with severe TD were treated with a mean clozapine dosage of 486 mg/day for 36 months. On follow-up at 100 weeks, 16 of the 30 patients showed a greater than 50% reduction of their TD symptoms on the Simpson Dyskinesia Scale, and 10 patients had complete remission. According to the investigators, symptoms did not reemerge over the follow-up period, suggesting a therapeutic effect of clozapine on TD that is distinct from neuroleptics that only mask the pathology. Lieberman's study seems to confirm the benefits of clozapine on TD from an earlier study by Gerbino et al. (1980).

Neuroleptic Malignant Syndrome

In rare instances, patients taking antipsychotic medications develop a potentially life-threatening disorder known as *neuroleptic malignant syndrome* or *NMS*. Although it occurs most frequently with the use of high-potency conventional antipsychotic drugs, this condition may appear during treatment with any antipsychotic agent, including atypical antipsychotics. Patients with NMS typically have marked muscle rigidity, although this feature may be absent in patients taking atypical antipsychotics. Other salient features include fever, autonomic instability, increased white blood cell (WBC) counts (>15,000/mm^3), increased creatine kinase levels (>300 U/mL), and delirium. The increased creatine kinase concentrations are the result of muscle breakdown, which can lead to myoglobinuria and acute renal failure.

Treatment includes discontinuation of the antipsychotic medication, administration of intravenous fluids and antipyretic agents, and use of cooling blankets. Dantrolene and bromocriptine improved symptoms of NMS in uncontrolled trials, but the drugs have not been shown to be more effective than supportive care. Bromocriptine is administered at an initial dosage of 1.25–2.5 mg twice daily, and the dosage may be increased to 10 mg three times a day (Guze and Baxter 1985). Dantrolene sodium, also used in the treatment of malignant hyperthermia (a rare reaction to anesthetic drugs), is a direct-acting muscle relaxant that may reduce the thermogenesis of NMS caused by the tonic contraction of skeletal muscles (Guze and Baxter 1985). The manufacturer's recommendation for administration of dantrolene for acute malignant hyperthermia is 1 mg/kg by rapid intravenous push. Administration of the drug should be continued until the symptoms are reversed or until a maximum dose of 10 mg/kg has been given. The oral dosage of dantrolene after a malignant hyperthermic crisis is 4–8 mg/kg/day in four divided doses. This regimen should be continued until all symptoms resolve. The potential for hepatotoxicity is significant with dantrolene therapy; thus, the drug should not be administered to patients with liver dysfunction.

Anticholinergic Side Effects

Anticholinergic side effects are categorized as peripheral or central. The most common peripheral side effects are dry mouth, decreased sweating, decreased bronchial secretions, blurred vision, difficulty with urination, constipation, and tachycardia. Bethanechol chloride, a cholinergic drug that does not cross the blood-brain barrier, may effectively treat these side effects at a dosage of 25–50 mg three times a day.

Central side effects of anticholinergic drugs include impairment in concentration, attention, and memory. These side effects must be differentiated from symptoms caused by the patient's psychosis. Some patients are subject to these symptoms at relatively low doses of medication. In cases of toxicity, anticholinergic delirium—which includes hot, dry skin; dry mucous membranes; dilated pupils; absent bowel sounds; tachycardia; and confusion—may occur. Anticholinergic delirium is a medical emergency, and full supportive medical care is required. Physostigmine, a centrally and peripherally acting reversible acetylcholinesterase, may be used as a diagnostic agent in cases of suspected anticholinergic toxicity. This agent is administered intramuscularly at a dose of 1–2 mg or intravenously at a slow controlled rate of no more than 1 mg/minute. Physostigmine should not be used to maintain reversal of the toxicity, however, because a cholinergic crisis may result, characterized by nausea, vomiting, bradycardia, and seizures. This reaction can be reversed by administering a potent anticholinergic drug such as atropine.

Adrenergic Side Effects

Antipsychotics block α_1-adrenergic receptors, which can result in orthostatic hypotension and dizziness. Administration of epinephrine, which stimulates both α- and β-adrenergic receptors, will result in a paradoxical decrease in blood pressure because of the stimulation of β-adrenergic receptors in the presence of α_1-adrenergic receptor blockade.

Weight Gain

Treatment with atypical antipsychotics is associated with a rapid increase in body weight during the first few months of therapy. Although the rate at which patients gain weight decreases with time, some patients continue to gain weight even after 1 year of treatment. Antipsychotics associated with weight gain include risperidone, quetiapine, chlorpromazine, thioridazine, olanzapine, and clozapine (Allison et al. 1999; American Diabetes Association et al. 2004). The amount of weight gained is not dose dependent and should be monitored throughout treatment.

Endocrine Effects and Sexual Side Effects

Numerous studies suggest a relation between the use of atypical antipsychotic medications and the development of hyperglycemia, dyslipidemia, and metabolic syndrome (American Diabetes Association et al. 2004; review by Citrome et al. 2005). The metabolic syndrome comprises a number of metabolic risk factors that may be associated with an increased cardiovascular risk. One definition of the metabolic syndrome specifies the presence of three or more of the five following clinical or laboratory features: 1) elevated plasma triglyceride levels ($\geq$150 mg/dL); 2) decreased plasma HDL levels (<50 mg/dL in women or <40 mg/dL in men); 3) elevated fasting glucose levels ($\geq$110 mg/dL); 4) waist circumference >35 inches in women or >40 inches in men; 5) elevated blood pressure ($\geq$130/85) (Citrome et al. 2005; Expert Panel on the Detection, Evaluation, and Treatment of High Blood Cholesterol in Adults 2001). Published guidelines recommend monitoring patients on atypical antipsychotics for several metabolic risk factors, including personal and family history of metabolic risks (baseline and annually), waist circumference (baseline and annually), body mass index (baseline, week 4, week 8, week 12, and quarterly), blood pressure and fasting glucose levels (baseline, week 12, and annually), and lipid panel (baseline, week 12, and every 5 years) (American Diabetes Association et al. 2004). Hyperglycemia can develop independent of or secondary to weight gain and, in some cases, resolves after discon-

tinuation of the medication. Patients taking clozapine and olanzapine have a higher risk of developing diabetes compared with patients taking other conventional and atypical antipsychotics (see American Diabetes Association et al. 2004). Data indicate that alterations in serum lipids are concordant with changes in body weight. Clozapine and olanzapine are associated with the greatest increases in total cholesterol, low-density lipoprotein, and triglycerides, as well as decreases in high-density lipoprotein. Aripiprazole and ziprasidone do not appear to be associated with dyslipidemia. Regardless, monitoring should be considered for all patients taking an antipsychotic medication.

All conventional antipsychotic medications and risperidone may cause hyperprolactinemia. Side effects mediated, at least in part, by hyperprolactinemia include gynecomastia, galactorrhea, amenorrhea, and decreased libido. Thioridazine may cause painful retrograde ejaculation.

Ocular Effects

Antipsychotics may cause pigmentary changes in the lens and retina, especially if the drugs are administered for long periods. Pigment deposition in the lens of the eye does not affect vision; however, pigmentary retinopathy, which can lead to irreversible blindness, has been associated specifically with the use of thioridazine. Although pigmentary retinopathy has most often been reported in patients taking more than 800 mg of thioridazine per day (the maximum recommended dose), this condition also has occurred at usual clinical doses (Ball and Caroff 1986; Hamilton 1985). Drug interactions may increase plasma levels of thioridazine, which may increase the risk of this dangerous side effect (Silver et al. 1986).

Quetiapine was associated with cataracts in preclinical safety studies conducted in beagles. Subsequent studies involving nonhuman primates did not detect an increased risk of cataracts; also, postmarketing surveys have not detected an increased risk of cataracts in patients taking quetiapine compared with patients taking other antipsychotics.

Dermatological Effects

Patients taking antipsychotics, especially the aliphatic phenothiazines (e.g., chlorpromazine), may become more sensitive to sunlight, which can lead to severe sunburn.

Cardiac Effects

In several studies, sudden death attributed to thioridazine or chlorpromazine therapy in young, healthy patients has been reported (Aherwadkar et al. 1974; Giles and Modlin 1968). Comparative trial data indicate that after the QT interval was corrected for heart rate, thioridazine produced the greatest mean delay in QTc (35.6 ms), followed by ziprasidone (20.6 ms), quetiapine (9.1 ms), olanzapine (6.8 ms), and haloperidol (4.7 ms) (data on file, U.S. Food and Drug Administration). Pimozide also may produce significant changes in cardiac conduction as a result of its calcium channel–blocking properties. It is recommended that serial electrocardiograms be performed when treatment with pimozide is started, and the drug should be discontinued if the QT interval exceeds 520 ms (in adults) or 470 ms (in children) (Baldessarini 1985). This strategy should be considered for patients taking thioridazine and ziprasidone, but it is not mandatory in healthy patients. Extremely high doses of intravenous haloperidol have been administered safely in patients with cardiac disease, although rare cases of torsades de pointes have been reported at these doses (Metzger and Friedman 1993). The cardiac effect of atypical antipsychotics in patients with underlying heart disease has not been adequately studied.

Hematological Effects

Agranulocytosis is an idiosyncratic reaction that usually occurs within the first 3–4 weeks of treatment with an antipsychotic drug. However, there is a continued risk, for 2–3 months, of agranulocytosis and leukopenia during treatment. A higher risk of agranulocytosis is associated with low-potency conventional antipsychotic drugs and, most significantly, clozapine. Signs and symptoms of this reaction include high fever, stomatitis, severe pharyngitis, lymphadenopathy, and malaise.

Lowered Seizure Threshold

Most conventional antipsychotics are associated with a dose-dependent risk of a lowered seizure threshold, although the incidence of seizures with most of these drugs is quite small (Devinsky et al. 1991). Of all the conventional antipsychotics, molindone and fluphenazine have been shown most consistently to have the lowest potential for this side effect (Itil and Soldatos 1980; Oliver et al. 1982). The atypical antipsychotic clozapine is associated with a dose-dependent risk of seizure.

Suppressed Temperature Regulation

Antipsychotic drugs directly affect the hypothalamus and suppress temperature regulation. Severe hyperthermia, rhabdomyolysis, renal failure, and death may result. A cool environment and adequate amounts of fluids are mandatory for patients taking antipsychotic agents.

Risks in Elderly Patients With Dementia

Treatment with atypical antipsychotics recently has been associated with an almost twofold increased mortality rate when used in elderly patients with dementia. Although these medications are not approved for treatment of dementia-related psychosis, such use is common in clinical practice (Herrmann and Lanctot 2005). At present, this appears to be a risk for the entire class. The risk associated with atypical antipsychotics is not statistically different from the risk associated with treatment with conventional antipsychotics (Gill et al. 2005).

■ DRUG INTERACTIONS

Antipsychotic drugs have profound effects on multiple central nervous system receptors, and these effects are compounded when other medications are added. For example, the α-adrenergic receptor blockade of antipsychotics may affect the efficacy of the antihypertensive drug guanethidine. The sedative and anticholinergic effects of antipsychotic drugs are increased with the addition of other sedating or anticholinergic drugs. As mentioned previously, patients taking drugs with potentially serious adverse effects (such as retinopathy associated with thioridazine) should be monitored through plasma level determinations when other medications are used concurrently.

Pharmacokinetic interactions with antipsychotic drugs are common and have been reviewed elsewhere (Goff and Baldessarini 1995). Most antipsychotics are metabolized by the hepatic cytochrome P450 (CYP) enzyme 2D6. Exceptions include ziprasidone and quetiapine, which are metabolized mainly by the CYP 3A4 enzyme. The activity of the 2D6 enzyme varies greatly (on the basis of genetic polymorphisms) among individuals and can be inhibited by certain drugs, such as selective serotonin reuptake inhibitors (SSRIs). For example, the addition of fluoxetine increased serum haloperidol concentrations by 20% and serum fluphenazine concentrations by 65% in one study (Goff et al 1995). Two categories of potential drug-drug interactions are of particular concern. The first includes interactions that can increase serum concentrations of antipsychotics to dangerous levels. For example, clozapine is metabolized by the CYP 2D6, 3A4, and 1A2 isoenzymes. When taken with CYP 3A4 and 1A2 inhibitors, such as erythromycin and fluvoxamine, serum clozapine concentrations can rise to toxic levels (Cohen et al. 1996; Wetzel et al. 1998). The other category of potentially serious interactions includes those that induce metabolism of antipsychotic agents, thereby lowering serum concentrations below a therapeutic threshold. Large reductions in serum clozapine and haloperidol concentrations have been reported with the addition of carbamazepine, phenobarbital, and phenytoin (Arana et al. 1986; Byerly and DeVane 1996). Of note, cigarette smoking can affect antipsychotic metabolism; serum concentrations of clozapine in particular are reduced with smoking and increased after smoking cessation (Byerly and DeVane 1996; Haring et al. 1989).

■ USE IN PREGNANCY

Like most other drugs, antipsychotic agents should be avoided, if possible, during pregnancy and during lactation (in the case of mothers who breast-feed their infants). The use of low-potency phenothiazine antipsychotics during the first trimester of pregnancy may increase the baseline risk of congenital anomalies by 0.4%, or 4 cases per 1,000 pregnancies (Altshuler et al. 1996). Less is known about the risks for teratogenicity, perinatal complications, and neurobehavioral problems associated with atypical antipsychotic medications. Thus far, retrospective studies, case reports, and clinical observations indicate that clozapine and olanzapine are not associated with an increased teratogenic risk. Data related to the use of aripiprazole, quetiapine, risperidone, and ziprasidone are still limited (see review by Gentile 2004). One case of agenesis of the corpus callosum was reported with risperidone use (Physicians' Desk Reference 2001). The use of medications in a woman who is pregnant is always a difficult decision. For example, the risk of fetal death is increased in psychotic mothers, so any risk of antipsychotic-induced teratogenesis must be assessed carefully and balanced against the risks involved in withholding treatment, both to the mother and to the fetus. Additionally, the risk for the development of hyperglycemia in conjunction with the use of atypical antipsychotic medications during pregnancy must be considered.

■ ATYPICAL ANTIPSYCHOTICS

Atypical antipsychotics cause fewer EPS than do conventional antipsychotics. Clozapine and quetiapine are the least likely to cause EPS and are therefore recommended for treatment of psychosis in patients with Parkinson's disease. With the notable exception of risperidone, atypical antipsychotics cause substantially less hyperprolactinemia than do conventional antipsychotics. Weight gain is a side effect of all atypical antipsychotics except ziprasidone and aripiprazole. Concerns about cardiac conduction delay with ziprasidone therapy exist and warrant consideration in patients who have risk factors for arrhythmias. Finally, sedation may be problematic with atypical antipsychotics, particularly with clozapine and quetiapine, and the risk of orthostatic hypotension necessitates careful titration of clozapine, quetiapine, and risperidone.

Aripiprazole

Aripiprazole is the most recently approved atypical antipsychotic. This medication has a high affinity for D_2 and D_3 receptors, as well as 5-HT_{1a} and 5-HT_{2a} receptors. Although the mechanism of action is not known, aripiprazole may mediate its effects via a combination of partial agonist activity at the D_2 and 5-HT_{1a} receptors and antagonist activity at the 5-HT_{2a} receptor.

Clinical Use

Aripiprazole has been approved for treatment of schizophrenia and acute manic or mixed episodes in bipolar disorder. This medication is also indicated for maintenance treatment in bipolar I disorder. The recommended starting and target dose for aripiprazole in patients with schizophrenia is 10 or 15 mg/day. This is a once-daily dose, and patients can take the medication with or without food. Although this medication has been shown to be effective in doses ranging from 10 to 30 mg/day, doses higher than 10–15 mg have not been shown to be more effective than 10- to 15-mg doses in patients with schizophrenia. The recommended starting dose for treatment of an acute manic or mixed episode is 30 mg; the recommended dose for maintenance treatment in stable patients is 15 mg/day. The elimination half-life is 75 hours, and steady-state concentrations are reached within 2 weeks. Therefore, dose adjustments are recommended every 2 weeks, to allow time for clinical assessments of the medication's effects to be observed at steady-state concentration. Peak plasma concentrations occur within 3–5 hours. At equivalent doses, the plasma concentrations of aripiprazole from the solution were higher compared with plasma concentrations associated with the tablet form.

Risks, Side Effects, and Their Management

The most common side effects associated with aripiprazole include headache, nausea, dyspepsia, agitation, anxiety, insomnia, somnolence, and akathisia. Dose-related adverse events include somnolence and akathisia. Early clinical experience indicates that akathisia may be avoided by starting the medication at doses lower than 10 mg and increasing the dose slowly. Aripiprazole is not associated with significant sedation, anticholinergic side effects, weight gain, or cardiovascular side effects (Petrie et al. 1997).

Drug Interactions

Aripiprazole is hepatically metabolized, mainly by two cytochrome P450 enzymes: CYP 2D6 and CYP 3A4. Therefore, dosage adjustments are necessary when this medication is given with other medications that either inhibit or induce these enzymes. For example, the dose of aripiprazole should be halved when this medication is given with ketoconazole, a CYP 3A4 inhibitor, or at least decreased when given with fluoxetine, a CYP 2D6 inhibitor. When aripiprazole is given with CYP 3A4 inducers such as carbamazepine, the dose should be doubled.

Clozapine

Clozapine, the first of the class of atypical antipsychotic drugs, rarely causes EPS, and it is the only antipsychotic drug that is not associated with treatment-emergent tardive dyskinesia. Because of the approximately 1% risk of potentially fatal agranulocytosis, the use of clozapine is restricted to patients who have not responded to or cannot tolerate other antipsychotic drugs.

Clinical Use

Because of prominent sedation and orthostatic hypotension, clozapine therapy is initiated at a dose of 12.5 mg/day, with a rapid increase to 12.5 mg twice a day. The dose is then increased as tolerated, generally in 25- or 50-mg increments every day or every other day. Clozapine is usually added to the previous antipsychotic agent in a cross-titration in which the dose of the previous drug is tapered once a clozapine dose of approximately 100 mg/day has been achieved. This strategy should be used with caution if the existing medication is a low-potency conventional antipsychotic because of the possibility of additive α-adrenergic and anticholinergic side effects. Clozapine doses can be increased much more rapidly in an inpatient setting, with monitoring of vital signs, than in an outpatient setting. The typical target dose is 300–500 mg/day in divided doses, with a greater amount given in the evening to minimize daytime sedation. Although routine blood level monitoring is not recommended, it should be noted that a serum level greater than 350 ng/mL is associated with a higher response rate (Perry et al. 1991). Serum levels should be ascertained in nonresponders. The oral disintegrating tablet is bioequivalent to the oral tablet.

The duration of treatment required to assess response is longer than for most medications—that is, typically 3–6 months (Meltzer 1994). The patient and the family must understand this time frame before clozapine therapy is initiated. If patients are nonresponsive after 6 months of continuous clozapine treatment, the dose may be gradually increased to a maximum of 900 mg/day. Not uncommonly, patients may not have significant reduction in symptoms with clozapine therapy, but review of their course over a 6-month or 1-year period shows a dramatic reduction in rates of relapse and hospitalization.

Risks, Side Effects, and Their Management

Agranulocytosis. Agranulocytosis was previously estimated to occur in 0.8% of patients receiving clozapine during the first year of treatment, with a peak incidence at 3 months (Alvir and Lieberman 1994; Alvir et al. 1993). The dispensing of clozapine in the United States is linked to weekly WBC counts during the first 6 months and biweekly counts thereafter. Strict guidelines based on WBC and absolute neutrophil counts have been set (Table 4–4). The system of hematological monitoring has reduced agranulocytosis-related fatalities to extremely low levels (Honigfeld et al. 1998).

TABLE 4–4. **Guidelines for hematological monitoring of patients taking clozapine**

1. Initial white blood cell (WBC) count must be greater than 3,500/mm^3, and absolute neutrophil count (ANC) must be greater than 2,000/mm^3.

2. Weekly WBC count and ANC are required for the first 6 months of treatment and for 4 weeks after discontinuation of clozapine. After 6 months, monitoring is required every 2 weeks; and after 12 months, monitoring is required every 4 weeks.

3. If WBC count is 2,000–3,000/mm^3 or ANC is 1,000–1,500/mm^3, interrupt therapy and monitor for signs of infection. Perform WBC and differential counts daily. If there are no symptoms of infection, if WBC count returns to greater than 3,000/mm^3, and if ANC is greater than 1,500/mm^3, resume clozapine therapy with twice-weekly WBC and differential counts until total WBC count returns to more than 3,500/mm^3 and ANC is greater than 2,000/mm^3.

4. If WBC count is less than 2,000/mm^3 or ANC is less than 1,000/mm^3, discontinue clozapine and do not rechallenge. Perform WBC and differential counts daily until WBC count is greater than 3,000/mm^3 and ANC is greater than 1,500/mm^3. Then monitor twice weekly until WBC count returns to more than 3,500/mm^3 and ANC is greater than 2,000/mm^3. Then monitor weekly for 4 weeks. Treat any infection with antibiotics. Consider bone marrow aspiration to ascertain granulopoietic status. If granulopoiesis is deficient, consider protective isolation.

Since the implementation of the Clozaril National Registry in the United States, the estimated rate of agranulocytosis has been estimated to be 0.38% on the basis of data collected from February 1990 to December 1994 (Honigfeld 1996; Honigfeld et al. 1998).

If agranulocytosis develops, prompt consultation with a hematologist is indicated. Reverse isolation and prophylactic antibiotics may be used to prevent infection. Granulocyte colony-stimulating factors may be used to shorten the duration of and reduce the morbidity of agranulocytosis (Barnas et al. 1992; Chengappa et al. 1996; Gerson et al. 1992; Nielsen 1993). Although lithium often causes leukocytosis, it does not appear to treat or prevent clozapine-induced agranulocytosis. Once a patient has developed agranulocytosis while taking clozapine, he or she should not be rechallenged with this medication.

Clozapine is contraindicated in patients who have myeloproliferative disorders or who are immunocompromised as a result of diseases such as active tuberculosis or human immunodeficiency virus infection because of their increased risk for agranulocytosis. Concomitant administration of medications that are associated with bone marrow suppression, such as carbamazepine, is also contraindicated.

Extrapyramidal side effects.   EPS are uncommon at any dose of clozapine, although some patients experience akathisia or hand tremors. There have been reports of NMS in patients medicated with clozapine alone (Anderson and Powers 1991; DasGupta and Young 1991; Miller et al. 1991).

Sedation.   Sedation is the most common side effect of clozapine, and it is particularly prominent early in treatment. Sedation generally attenuates when the dose is reduced, when tolerance to this side effect develops, or when a disproportionate amount is given at bedtime.

Cardiovascular effects.   Hypotension and tachycardia occur in most patients taking clozapine. Cases of potentially fatal myocarditis and dilated cardiomyopathy have been reported in association with clozapine (Kilian et al. 1999). Myocarditis typically occurred within 3 weeks of starting clozapine, but cardiomyopathy may not be apparent for several years. Although rare, treatment-emergent myocarditis and cardiomyopathy occur at a reportedly higher incidence with clozapine than with other antipsychotics (Coulter et al. 2001). The mechanism by which clozapine may cause myocarditis has not been established, but some authors have speculated that clozapine may cause an immunoglobulin E (IgE)-mediated type I hypersensitivity reaction (Kilian et al. 1999) or a hypereosinophilic syndrome (Hagg et al. 2001).

Weight gain.   Weight gain occurs in most patients; body weight increases by 10% or more in many patients (Umbricht et al. 1994).

One naturalistic study found that weight gain did not plateau with clozapine therapy until year 4, and the weight gain was not dose related (Henderson et al. 2000). Patients should receive nutritional counseling at the initiation of treatment with clozapine.

Hypersalivation.   Hypersalivation occurs in one-third of the patients taking clozapine (it occurs particularly at night).

Fever.   For unclear reasons, clozapine is associated with benign, transient temperature increases, generally within the first 3 weeks of treatment. Patients taking clozapine who develop fevers should be evaluated for infections, agranulocytosis, and NMS.

Seizures.   Clozapine is associated with a dose-dependent risk of seizures. The vast majority of clozapine-induced seizures are tonic-clonic, but myoclonic seizures also occur. Doses less than 300 mg/day are associated with a 1% risk of seizures. Doses of 300–600 mg/day carry a 2.7% risk, and doses greater than 600 mg/day are associated with a 4.4% risk (Devinsky et al. 1991). Because of this risk, clozapine doses greater than 600 mg/day are not recommended unless the patient's symptoms have not responded at lower doses. Many clinicians avoid administering clozapine to patients with abnormal electroencephalographic findings. Our clinical impression is that electroencephalographic abnormalities associated with clozapine use are much more common than clozapine-induced seizures. Once a seizure has occurred, determining whether to continue using clozapine requires clinical judgment. Because only patients with fairly serious and otherwise refractory illnesses receive clozapine, treatment with this medication is usually continued, with the addition of an anticonvulsant. Carbamazepine must be avoided because of the additive risk of bone marrow suppression. At present, valproate appears to be the safest anticonvulsant for patients taking clozapine.

Anticholinergic side effects.   Anticholinergic effects, such as dry mouth, blurred vision, constipation, and urinary retention, are common early side effects.

Obsessive-compulsive symptoms.   Clozapine has been reported to exacerbate symptoms of obsessive-compulsive disorder, probably because of 5-HT$_2$ antagonism (Ghaemi et al. 1995). If this effect occurs, symptoms are usually controlled with the addition of an SSRI.

Drug Interactions

Clozapine should not be combined with any drugs that have the potential to suppress bone marrow function, such as carbamazepine. There have been isolated reports of respiratory arrest in patients taking both clozapine and a high-potency benzodiazepine. Thus, benzodiazepines (particularly in high doses) should not be administered to patients taking clozapine.

Clozapine is metabolized by hepatic CYP 1A2 and, to a lesser degree, CYP 3A3/4; therefore, the drug is subject to changes in serum concentration when combined with medications that inhibit or induce these enzymes. Serum clozapine levels increase with coadministration of fluvoxamine or erythromycin and decrease with coadministration of phenobarbital or phenytoin and with cigarette smoking (Byerly and DeVane 1996). These pharmacokinetic interactions are particularly important because of the dose-dependent risk of seizures.

Risperidone

Risperidone, a novel benzisoxazole derivative, is an atypical antipsychotic medication that combines dopamine D$_2$ receptor antagonism with potent 5-HT$_2$ receptor antagonism. Risperidone has a higher affinity for dopamine D$_2$ receptors than does clozapine. Risperidone also antagonizes dopamine D$_1$ and D$_4$ receptors, α_1- and α_2-adrenergic receptors, and histamine H$_1$ receptors. Although the optimal dose of risperidone in North American trials was 6 mg/day, subsequent clinical experience has indicated that most patients do well at lower doses of 3–6 mg/day, and elderly patients may require doses as low as 0.5 mg/day. Unlike other atypical antipsychotics, risperidone increases prolactin levels; these levels are often higher than those associated with conventional antipsychotics.

Clinical Use

Risperidone is most effective at 4- to 6-mg doses. For initial treatment, we recommend using divided doses, starting at 1 mg twice a day and quickly increasing to 2 mg twice a day. For elderly persons, the initial dose should be much lower (0.25–0.5 mg/day). After the first week of treatment, the entire dose can be given at bedtime. This approach usually helps the patient sleep and reduces daytime side effects. However, we do not suggest this practice for elderly persons because of an increased risk of falling. In some patients, risperidone has an activating effect; these individuals should take the medication in the morning. All three oral forms of this medication are bioequivalent.

Risperidone is the only atypical antipsychotic currently available in a long-acting injectable form (Risperdal Consta). Details regarding dosing strategies are discussed earlier in this chapter. Results from a 12-week, multicenter, double-blind study indicate that long-acting risperidone is more effective than placebo for improving the positive and negative symptoms associated with schizophrenia (Kane et al. 2003). According to numerous studies, the medication is well tolerated (Fleischhacker et al. 2003; Kane et al. 2003). Thus far, no randomized controlled trials have compared the long-acting injectable form of risperidone with depot preparations of typical antipsychotics.

Risks, Side Effects, and Their Management

Insomnia, hypotension, agitation, headache, and rhinitis are the most common side effects of risperidone. These tend to lessen with time. Overall, the drug tends to be well tolerated. Average weight gain associated with risperidone after 10 weeks of treatment is 2.10 kg (Allison et al. 1999). Risperidone does not have significant anticholinergic side effects. Hyperprolactinemia is common.

Cardiovascular effects. Brief hypotension may occur, as may be expected with α-adrenergic receptor blockade. Tachycardia is also common.

Drug Interactions

Risperidone is metabolized primarily by CYP 2D6 (Byerly and De-Vane 1996). Medications that inhibit this enzyme, such as many of the SSRIs, cause increases in plasma risperidone levels. Pharmacodynamic interactions may occur when risperidone is combined with medications that share a similar physiological effect, such as orthostatic hypotension.

Olanzapine

Like risperidone, olanzapine is a selective monoaminergic antagonist with high-affinity binding at the 5-HT_2 and D_1, D_2, D_3, and D_4 receptors.

Clinical Use

The recommended starting dosage of olanzapine is 10 mg at bedtime for patients with schizophrenia and 10–15 mg qhs for acutely manic patients. The clinically effective dose range is 7.5–20 mg/day (5–20 mg/day in mania), and a single daily dose is administered at bedtime. Higher doses may be required in some patients. Clinically meaningful improvement may not be evident for the first several weeks after initiation of treatment. Usual doses for maintenance treatment in patients with bipolar disorder range from 5 mg to 20 mg daily. Pharmacokinetic studies show that the oral disintegrating tablet and the solution form of the medication are bioequivalent to the tablet. Although no systematic data are available regarding switching from other antipsychotic drugs to olanzapine, early clinical experience favors a gradual cross-titration. Commonly, olanzapine is added to the existing antipsychotic medication, whose dose is tapered after 1–2 weeks.

Olanzapine is also available in a short-acting intramuscular injectable form, providing clinicians with another option for treating acute agitation associated with psychosis or mania. A double-blind, placebo-controlled comparison of intramuscular olanzapine and intramuscular haloperidol in the treatment of acute agitation in patients with schizophrenia indicated that treatment with olanzapine was superior to intramuscular placebo injections for decreasing agitation; this reduction in agitation was dose dependent. No significant difference in response was seen between the haloperidol and the olanzapine groups. Olanzapine was well tolerated (Breier et al. 2002). Peak plasma concentrations are achieved within 15–45 minutes. It is available in vials containing 10 mg of olanzapine for administration.

Risks, Side Effects, and Their Management

Somnolence.   As one would expect, given the histamine H_1 receptor antagonism, somnolence is a common side effect of olanzapine. Somnolence and psychomotor slowing are dose dependent, and patients often become tolerant to this side effect over time.

Anticholinergic side effects.   Anticholinergic side effects are clinically less significant than would be predicted on the basis of in vitro muscarinic receptor–binding affinity. However, dry mouth may occur.

Seizures.   Treatment-emergent seizures are rare in the absence of concomitant medical disorders. Olanzapine should be used with caution in patients with a history of seizures and in patients with conditions that may lower the seizure threshold, such as dementia.

Hepatic effects.   Increased transaminase levels occur in approximately 2% of the patients taking olanzapine. In many cases, these levels normalize without medication discontinuation, and all cases to date have been clinically benign. Routine laboratory monitoring is not recommended, but olanzapine should be used with caution in patients with hepatic disease or with additional risk factors for hepatic toxicity. In this group of patients, serum transaminase levels must be monitored.

Weight gain.   Treatment-emergent weight gain is common with olanzapine therapy and averages about 4.15 kg after 10 weeks of treatment (Allison et al. 1999). By 39 weeks, weight gain tends to plateau (Kinon et al. 2001), and approximately 20% of patients may not gain weight. Patients with higher body mass indices (>27.6 kg/m^2) tend to gain less weight than do those with lower body mass indices. Weight gain is independent of dose (Kinon et al. 2001).

Drug Interactions

Olanzapine is metabolized by several pathways and is therefore unlikely to be affected by concurrent administration of other medications. Because olanzapine does not appear to inhibit any cytochrome P450 enzymes, it should not increase the availability of other medications through inhibition of such enzymes. Additive pharmacodynamic effects are expected if olanzapine is combined with medications that also have anticholinergic, antihistaminic, or α_1-adrenergic side effects.

Quetiapine

The receptor properties of quetiapine are similar to those for olanzapine and risperidone. This medication is rapidly absorbed, reaching peak plasma concentrations in 1.5 hours. It is metabolized by the liver.

Clinical Use

Quetiapine is indicated for the treatment of schizophrenia and acute mania. Results from a recent study also showed that this medication is an effective treatment for bipolar depression (Calabrese et al. 2005). Quetiapine therapy is initiated at a dose of 25 mg twice a day for patients with schizophrenia, with increases to 50 mg twice a day on day 2, 100 mg twice a day on day 3, and 100 mg in the morning and 200 mg in the evening on day 4. The optimal dose for most patients appears to range between 400 and 600 mg/day, although the drug is safe and efficacious for some patients within a dose range of

150–750 mg. Slower titration and lower daily doses may be warranted in patients with hepatic disease and in elderly patients. Because of its relatively short half-life of 6–8 hours, quetiapine is usually administered twice daily.

For patients who have acute mania, treatment should be initiated with twice-daily doses totaling 100 mg on day 1, 200 mg on day 2, 300 mg on day 3, and 400 mg on day 4. Additional adjustments up to 800 mg/day by day 6 can be made. Doses should not be increased by more than 200 mg/day on days 5 and 6. Most patients respond to doses between 400 and 800 mg/day.

Risks, Side Effects, and Their Management

In terms of EPS and changes in serum prolactin levels, quetiapine at doses of up to 750 mg/day was no different from placebo (Arvanitis and Miller 1997).

Somnolence. Somnolence is one of the most common side effects of quetiapine. Somnolence and psychomotor slowing are dose dependent, and patients often become tolerant to these side effects over time.

Ocular changes. Cataracts developed in association with quetiapine treatment in preclinical studies involving dogs, but a causal relation has not been established in humans. Postmarketing trials have not detected an increase in the incidence of cataracts with quetiapine compared with other antipsychotics.

Cardiovascular effects. Given α_1-adrenergic receptor antagonism, quetiapine may induce orthostatic hypotension and concomitant symptoms of dizziness, tachycardia, and syncope. The risk of symptomatic hypotension is particularly pronounced during initial dose titration. Quetiapine should be used with caution in patients with cardiovascular disease, cerebrovascular disease, or other illnesses predisposing to hypotension.

Hepatic effects. In premarketing trials, increased transaminase levels were noted in 6% of patients taking quetiapine. These changes usually occur in the first weeks of treatment and to date have been benign. Routine laboratory monitoring is not recommended, but quetiapine should be used with caution in patients with hepatic disease or with additional risk factors for hepatic toxicity.

Weight gain.   Quetiapine is associated with weight gain. In premarketing placebo-controlled studies, a weight gain of at least 7% of body weight was observed in 23% of the quetiapine-treated patients with schizophrenia, compared with 6% of the control subjects given placebo. Similar findings were observed in placebo-controlled trials of mania monotherapy (Seroquel 2005).

Drug Interactions

Quetiapine is metabolized by hepatic CYP 3A3/4. Concurrent administration of cytochrome P450–inducing drugs, such as carbamazepine, decreases blood levels of quetiapine. In such circumstances, increased doses of quetiapine are appropriate. Quetiapine does not appreciably affect the pharmacokinetics of other medications. Pharmacodynamic effects are expected if quetiapine is combined with medications that also have antihistaminic or α-adrenergic side effects. Because of its potential for inducing hypotension, quetiapine also may enhance the effects of certain antihypertensive agents.

Ziprasidone

Ziprasidone is the only atypical antipsychotic available in capsule form. Like risperidone, quetiapine, and olanzapine, it is a 5-HT$_{2a}$ and D$_2$ antagonist.

Clinical Use

Ziprasidone is approved for the treatment of schizophrenia and acute mania. For patients with schizophrenia, ziprasidone is usually started at a dosage of 20–40 mg twice a day. In medically healthy, nonelderly patients, the dose can be rapidly titrated over 2–4 days to a typical therapeutic dosage of 60–80 mg twice a day. For patients with acute mania, treatment should be initiated at 40 mg twice a day. This dose should be increased to 60 or 80 mg on day 2 and subsequently adjusted on the basis of individual tolerance and symptoms to between 40 and 80 mg twice a day. Ziprasidone has a half-life of 5–10 hours and is usually administered twice daily with meals. Food increases absorption by approximately 100%. Because safety data regarding ziprasidone are largely derived from studies that exclude subjects with cardiac disease, clinicians should screen patients (preferably with a baseline electrocardiogram and measurement of serum electrolyte levels) for cardiac risk factors before initiating ziprasidone therapy. Patients with QTc prolongation at baseline must be monitored very closely; a cardiology consultation is recommended.

The recommended dose for intramuscular injection (for the treatment of acute agitation associated with schizophrenia) is 10–20 mg, with a maximum dose of 40 mg/day. The 10-mg doses can be administered every 2 hours, whereas the 20-mg doses can be administered every 4 hours. Peak plasma concentrations are achieved by 60 minutes.

Risks, Side Effects, and Their Management

The most common side effects are headache, dyspepsia, nausea, constipation, abdominal pain, somnolence, and EPS. Ratings of parkinsonism and akathisia with ziprasidone, 120 mg/day, did not differ from those with placebo. Although dizziness has been reported, rates of orthostatic hypotension have not differed from rates associated with placebo in controlled clinical trials.

Cardiovascular side effects. Ziprasidone produced a mean QTc prolongation of 21 ms at maximal blood levels achieved with typical therapeutic doses. However, in all clinical trials, the rate of QTc intervals greater than 500 ms (considered a threshold for arrhythmia risk) did not differ from the rate associated with placebo (<0.1%). The QTc effect of ziprasidone is larger than that of other atypical antipsychotics but smaller than that of thioridazine. Blood levels of ziprasidone increased about 40% when ketoconazole (a metabolic inhibitor) was coadministered, and no change in QTc duration was detected.

Weight gain.   Ziprasidone is associated with less weight gain than are other atypical antipsychotic agents.

Drug Interactions

Drugs that inhibit CYP 3A4 reduce metabolism of ziprasidone: concurrent treatment with ketoconazole increased blood levels of ziprasidone by approximately 40%. Carbamazepine (and possibly other enzyme inducers) may decrease ziprasidone levels by approximately 35%. Effects of ziprasidone on metabolism of other drugs have not been reported.

■ CONVENTIONAL ANTIPSYCHOTICS

Atypical antipsychotics have replaced conventional antipsychotics as first-line treatments for schizophrenia. Drug potency is a useful construct for comparing conventional antipsychotics and their side-effect profiles. The term *drug potency* refers to the milligram equivalence of drugs, not to the relative efficacy. For example, although haloperidol is more potent than chlorpromazine (haloperidol 2 mg = chlorpromazine 100 mg), therapeutically equivalent doses are equally effective (haloperidol 12 mg = chlorpromazine 600 mg). Typically, the potency of antipsychotic drugs is compared with the potency of 100 mg of chlorpromazine. As a rule, high-potency conventional antipsychotics have an equivalent dose of less than 5 mg (Table 4–1). These medications are associated with more EPS but less sedation, fewer anticholinergic side effects, and less hypotension. Low-potency conventional antipsychotic drugs have an equivalent dose of more than 40 mg. These drugs are associated with greater sedation, more anticholinergic side effects, and more hypotension; however, acute EPS are less frequent. Tardive dyskinesia rates for high- and low-potency conventional antipsychotics do not differ. Antipsychotic drugs with intermediate potency (i.e., an equivalent dose between 5 and 40 mg) have a side-effect profile that lies between the profiles of these two groups. In most circumstances in which conventional antipsychotics are used, high-potency drugs are preferred because EPS usually can be minimized by using the lowest effective dose or by treating symptomatically, whereas anticholinergic and autonomic side effects are potentially more dangerous and difficult to manage. Intermediate-potency conventional antipsychotics are sometimes useful in patients who cannot tolerate high- or low-potency drugs.

■ LONG-ACTING INJECTABLE ANTIPSYCHOTICS

For patients with chronic psychotic symptoms who do not comply with a daily medication regimen, a long-acting depot preparation should be considered after stabilization with oral medication. Fluphenazine, haloperidol, and risperidone are the only long-acting injectable antipsychotic medications currently available in the United States.

Conversion to a decanoate preparation is complicated by the highly variable individual pharmacokinetics of the oral and long-term depot agents. Most patients respond to a fluphenazine decanoate dose of 10–30 mg given every 2 weeks (Baldessarini et al. 1988). A loading dose strategy has been established for haloperidol decanoate, in which patients receive an initial dose that is 20 times the oral maintenance dose (Ereshefsky et al. 1993). The maximum volume per injection of haloperidol decanoate should not exceed 3 mL, and the maximum dose per injection should not exceed 100 mg. If 20 times the oral dose is greater than 100 mg, the dose is given in divided injections spaced 3–7 days apart. Subsequent doses are decreased monthly, to about 10 times the oral dose by the third or fourth month. Ten times the oral dose, administered every 4 weeks, is a typical maintenance dose for haloperidol decanoate. For elderly or debilitated patients, the initial dose is 10–15 times the previous oral daily dose. Many clinicians prefer to continue giving oral medication at approximately half the previous maintenance dose during the first few months of depot antipsychotic administration rather than administer a loading dose of depot medication. This approach allows greater flexibility with regard to initial dose titration. In either approach, breakthrough psychotic symptoms are treated with supplemental oral medication, and the dose of the next scheduled depot injection can be increased accordingly. Steady-state serum concentrations are achieved after approximately 10 weeks (five injection intervals) with fluphenazine decanoate and after approximately 20 weeks with haloperidol decanoate. Side effects may take months to subside, and withdrawal dyskinesia may not appear for months after discontinuation of the decanoate formulation.

The recommended starting dose for the risperidone long-acting injection is 25 mg regardless of the patient's previous or current oral dose of antipsychotic medication. Although an initial release of medication occurs, the amount released is small, and the main release of the drug starts from 3 weeks after the injection onward. This release is maintained from 4 to 6 weeks and subsides by 7 weeks. Because not much drug is released for the first 3 weeks after the injection, oral antipsychotic supplementation is recommended. Injections are given every 2 weeks, and steady-state plasma concentrations are achieved after four injections. Dosing adjustments should not be made more often than once a month; the maximum dose is 50 mg every 2 weeks. Doses of 25, 37.5, and 50 mg are available, and different dosage strengths should not be combined. Dose titration depends on clinical symptoms. If the patient has not taken risperidone before, a trial of oral risperidone is recommended to determine whether the patient has a hypersensitivity reaction to the medication.

■ TREATMENT OF SCHIZOPHRENIA

General Principles

Evidence indicates that the long-term outcome for a patient with schizophrenia is better when treatment of the acute episode is initiated rapidly. After a patient's first psychotic episode, treatment with the antipsychotic medication should be continued for at least 1 year after a full remission of psychotic symptoms. A trial period without medication may then be considered, except for patients with a history of serious suicide attempts or violent aggressive behavior

(Lehman et al. 2004). The patient and his or her family should be informed about the early signs and symptoms of relapse, such as suspiciousness, difficulty sleeping, and argumentativeness, and should be warned that relapse is highly likely. Some evidence shows that first-episode psychosis may be more responsive to treatment and require lower doses of antipsychotic medications compared with patients with multiple prior psychotic episodes (Lieberman et al. 1996, 1998; McEvoy et al. 1991; Schooler et al. 1997; Zhang-Wong et al. 1999), although the time to response may be longer (Lieberman et al. 1993). Additionally, a longer duration of illness prior to treatment may be a predictor of poorer treatment response and a longer time to remission (Loebel et al. 1992). These data suggest that initiating treatment early, starting with low antipsychotic doses, and allowing adequate time (e.g., 2–4 weeks) for response may be the preferred approach with these patients.

The 2004 "Practice Guideline for the Treatment of Patients With Schizophrenia" recommends indefinite maintenance treatment for patients who have had at least two episodes of psychosis within 5 years or who have had multiple previous episodes (Lehman et al. 2004). Maintenance therapy should involve the lowest possible doses of antipsychotic drugs, and patients should be monitored closely for symptoms of relapse. If the patient is compliant with treatment, oral medications are usually sufficient. However, if the patient's treatment history suggests that the patient may not reliably take daily oral medication, a long-acting depot preparation may be indicated.

Treatment-Resistant Schizophrenia

If the schizophrenic symptoms are not responding to the indicated treatment, if the patient is experiencing minimal side effects (e.g., EPS, hypotension, sedation), and if poor compliance is not the cause, the physician can gradually increase the dose until mild side effects are noted. If no further improvement is seen after an additional 2–4 weeks at this dose, a different antipsychotic should be started. Usually, treatment with more than one atypical antipsychotic is tried before a conventional antipsychotic medication is started. A trial of clozapine should be considered for patients who have not responded to adequate trials of other antipsychotic medications. Electroconvulsive therapy should be considered for patients with catatonia, suicidal ideation or behavior, or persistent severe psychosis or for whom previous treatments, including clozapine, have not been effective (Lehman et al. 2004).

An additional strategy to use in nonresponsive patients is to add another medication to augment the therapeutic effects of the antipsychotic. Current augmentation strategies include adding an anticonvulsant, another antipsychotic, a benzodiazepine, or a cholinergic agent (Lehman et al. 2004). Different medications may help target specific symptoms, such as affective lability, aggression, or anxiety. Augmentation with an SSRI may be helpful for depressive symptoms and for negative symptoms, although clinicians should monitor patients carefully for pharmacokinetic interactions (Evins and Goff 1996). Although no systematic data are available to guide the treatment of schizophrenia that has not responded to clozapine, some patients may benefit from the combination of clozapine and another atypical antipsychotic (Henderson and Goff 1996). Because of the potential side effects and added cost, combination therapy should be attempted only after an adequate trial of monotherapy. The combination of cognitive-behavioral therapy and medication in patients with refractory schizophrenia is helpful (Lehman et al. 2004).

■ REFERENCES

Aherwadkar SJ, Efendigil MC, Coulshed N: Chlorpromazine therapy and associated acute disturbances of cardiac rhythm. Br Heart J 36:1251–1252, 1974

Allison DB, Mentore JL, Heo M, et al: Antipsychotic-induced weight gain: a comprehensive research synthesis. Am J Psychiatry 156:1686–1696, 1999

Altshuler LL, Cohen L, Szuba MP, et al: Pharmacologic management of psychiatric illness during pregnancy: dilemmas and guidelines. Am J Psychiatry 153:592–606, 1996

Alvir JM, Lieberman JA: Agranulocytosis: incidence and risk factors. J Clin Psychiatry 55 (suppl B):137–138, 1994

Alvir JM, Lieberman JA, Safferman AZ, et al: Clozapine-induced agranulo-cytosis: incidence and risk factors in the United States. N Engl J Med 329:162–167, 1993

American Diabetes Association, American Psychiatric Association, American Association of Clinical Endocrinologists, North American Association for the Study of Obesity: Consensus development conference on antipsychotic drugs and obesity and diabetes. Diabetes Care 27:596–601, 2004

American Psychiatric Association: Tardive Dyskinesia: A Task Force Report of the American Psychiatric Association. Washington, DC, American Psychiatric Association, 1992

Anderson ES, Powers PS: Neuroleptic malignant syndrome associated with clozapine use. J Clin Psychiatry 52:102–104, 1991

Arana GW, Goff DC, Friedman H, et al: Does carbamazepine-induced reduction of plasma haloperidol levels worsen psychotic symptoms? Am J Psychiatry 143:650–651, 1986

Arvanitis LA, Miller BG: Multiple fixed doses of "Seroquel" (quetiapine) in patients with acute exacerbation of schizophrenia: a comparison with haloperidol and placebo. The Seroquel Trial 13 Study Group. Biol Psychiatry 42:233–246, 1997

Baldessarini RJ: Chemotherapy in Psychiatry: Principles and Practice. Cambridge, MA, Harvard University Press, 1985

Baldessarini RJ, Cohen BM, Teicher MH: Significance of neuroleptic dose and plasma level in the pharmacological treatment of psychoses. Arch Gen Psychiatry 45:79–91, 1988

Ball WA, Caroff SN: Retinopathy, tardive dyskinesia, and low-dose thioridazine (letter). Am J Psychiatry 143:256–257, 1986

Barnas C, Zwierzina H, Hummer M, et al: Granulocyte-macrophage colony-stimulating factor (GM-CSF) treatment of clozapine-induced agranulo-cytosis: a case report. J Clin Psychiatry 53:245–247, 1992

Breier A, Meehan K, Birkett M, et al: A double-blind, placebo-controlled dose-response comparison of intramuscular olanzapine and haloperidol in the treatment of acute agitation in schizophrenia. Arch Gen Psychiatry 59:441–448, 2002

Byerly MJ, DeVane CL: Pharmacokinetics of clozapine and risperidone: a review of recent literature. J Clin Psychopharmacol 16:177–187, 1996

Calabrese JR, Keck PE, Macfadden W, et al: A randomized, double-blind, placebo-controlled trial of quetiapine in the treatment of bipolar I or II depression. Am J Psychiatry 162:1351–1360, 2005

Chengappa KN, Gopalani A, Haught MK, et al: The treatment of clozapine-associated agranulocytosis with granulocyte colony-stimulating factor (G-CSF). Psychopharmacol Bull 32:111–121, 1996

Citrome L, Blonde L, Damatarca C: Metabolic issues in patients with severe mental illness. South Med J 98:714–720, 2005

Cohen LG, Chesley S, Eugenio L, et al: Erythromycin-induced clozapine toxic reaction. Arch Intern Med 156:675–677, 1996

Correll CU, Leucht S, Kane JM: Lower risk for tardive dyskinesia associated with second generation antipsychotics: a systematic review of 1-year studies. Am J Psychiatry 161:414–425, 2004

Coulter DM, Bate A, Meyboom RHB, et al: Antipsychotic drugs and heart muscle disorder in international pharmacovigilance: data mining study. BMJ 222:1207–1209, 2001

DasGupta K, Young A: Clozapine-induced neuroleptic malignant syndrome. J Clin Psychiatry 52:105–107, 1991

Davis KL, Kahn RS, Ko G, et al: Dopamine in schizophrenia: a review and reconceptualization. Am J Psychiatry 148:1474–1486, 1991

Devinsky O, Honigfeld G, Patin J: Clozapine-related seizures. Neurology 41:369–371, 1991

Ereshefsky L, Toney G, Saklad SR, et al: A loading-dose strategy for converting from oral to depot haloperidol. Hosp Community Psychiatry 44:1155–1161, 1993

Evins A, Goff D: Adjunctive antidepressant drug therapies in the treatment of negative symptoms of schizophrenia. CNS Drugs 6:130–147, 1996

Expert Panel on the Detection, Evaluation, and Treatment of High Blood Cholesterol in Adults: executive summary of the third report of the National Cholesterol Education Program (NCEP) expert panel on detection, evaluation, and treatment of high blood cholesterol in adults (Adult Treatment Panel III). JAMA 285:2486–2497, 2001

Fleischhacker WW, Eerdekens M, Karcher K, et al: Treatment of schizophrenia with long-acting injectable risperidone: a 12-month open label trial of the first long-acting second-generation antipsychotic. J Clin Psychiatry 64:1250–1257, 2003

Fuller MA, Sajatovic M: Drug Information Handbook for Psychiatry, 4th Edition. Hudson, OH, Lexi-Comp, 2004, pp 1440–1441

Gentile S: Clinical utilization of atypical antipsychotics in pregnancy and lactation. Ann Pharmacother 38:1265–1271, 2004

Gerbino L, Shopsin B, Collora M: Clozapine in the treatment of tardive dyskinesia: an interim report, in Tardive Dyskinesia, Research and Treatment. Edited by Fann WE, Smith RC, Davis JM, et al. New York, SP Medical and Scientific Books, 1980, pp 475–489

Gerson SL, Gullion G, Yeh HS, et al: Granulocyte colony-stimulating factor for clozapine-induced agranulocytosis (letter). Lancet 340:1097, 1992

Ghaemi SN, Zarate CA Jr, Popli AP, et al: Is there a relationship between clozapine and obsessive-compulsive disorder? A retrospective chart review. Compr Psychiatry 36:267–270, 1995

Giles TD, Modlin RK: Death associated with ventricular arrhythmia and thioridazine hydrochloride. JAMA 205:108–110, 1968

Gill SS, Rochon PA, Herrmann N, et al: Atypical antipsychotic drugs and risk of ischaemic stroke: population based retrospective cohort study. BMJ 330:445, 2005 (Epub January 24, 2005)

Glazer WM, Moore DC, Schooler NR, et al: Tardive dyskinesia: a discontinuation study. Arch Gen Psychiatry 41:623–627, 1984

Goff D[C], Baldessarini R: Antipsychotics, in Drug Interactions in Psychiatry, 2nd Edition. Edited by Ciraulo D, Shader R, Greenblatt D, et al. Baltimore, MD, Williams & Wilkins, 1995, pp 129–174

Goff DC, Evins AE: Negative symptoms in schizophrenia: neurobiological models and treatment response. Harv Rev Psychiatry 6:59–77, 1998

Goff DC, Midha KK, Sarid-Segal O, et al: A placebo-controlled trial of fluoxetine added to neuroleptic in patients with schizophrenia. Psychopharmacology (Berl) 117:417–423, 1995

Guze BH, Baxter LR: Current concepts: neuroleptic malignant syndrome. N Engl J Med 313:163–166, 1985

Hagg S, Spigset O, Bate A, et al: Myocarditis related to clozapine treatment. J Clin Psychopharmacol 21:382–388, 2001

Hamilton JD: Thioridazine retinopathy within the upper dosage limit. Psychosomatics 26:823–824, 1985

Haring C, Barnas C, Saria A, et al: Dose-related plasma levels of clozapine. J Clin Psychopharmacol 9:71–72, 1989

Henderson DC, Goff DC: Risperidone as an adjunct to clozapine therapy in chronic schizophrenics. J Clin Psychiatry 57:395–397, 1996

Henderson DC, Cagliero E, Gray C, et al: Clozapine, diabetes mellitus, weight gain, and lipid abnormalities: a five year naturalistic study. Am J Psychiatry 157:975–981, 2000

Herrmann N, Lanctot KL: Do atypical antipsychotics cause stroke? CNS Drugs 19:91–103, 2005

Honigfeld G: The Clozapine National Registry System: forty years of risk management. J Clin Psychiatry Monogr 14:29–32, 1996

Honigfeld G, Arellano F, Sethi J, et al: Reducing clozapine-related morbidity and mortality: 5 years of experience with the Clozaril National Registry. J Clin Psychiatry 59 (suppl 3):3–7, 1998

Itil TM, Soldatos C: Epileptogenic side effects of psychotropic drugs: practical recommendations. JAMA 244:1460–1463, 1980

Jeste DV, Lacro JP, Bailey A, et al: Lower incidence of tardive dyskinesia with risperidone compared to haloperidol in older patients. J Am Geriatr Soc 47:716–719, 1999

Kane JM, Eerdekens M, Lindenmayer JP, et al: Long-acting injectable risperidone: efficacy and safety of the first long-acting atypical antipsychotic. Am J Psychiatry 160:1125–1132, 2003

Kilian JG, Kerr K, Lawrence C, et al. Myocarditis and cardiomyopathy associated with clozapine. Lancet 354:1841–1845, 1999

Kinon BJ, Basson BR, Gilmore JA, et al: Long-term olanzapine treatment: weight change and weight-related health factors in schizophrenia. J Clin Psychiatry 62:92–100, 2001

Kiuchi K, Hirata Y, Minami M, et al: Effect of 7-{3-[4-(2,3-dimethylphenyl)piperazinyl]propoxy}-2(1H)-quinolinone (OPC-4392), a newly synthesized agonist for presynaptic dopamine D_2 receptor, on tyrosine hydroxylation in rat striatal slices. Life Sci 42:343–349, 1988

Lehman AF, Lieberman JA, Dixon LB, et al: Practice guideline for the treatment of patients with schizophrenia, second edition. Am J Psychiatry 161 (suppl 2):1–56, 2004

Lieberman JA: Atypical antipsychotic drugs as a first-line treatment of schizophrenia: a rationale and hypothesis. J Clin Psychiatry 57 (suppl 11):68–71, 1996

Lieberman JA, Saltz BL, Johns CA, et al: The effects of clozapine on tardive dyskinesia. Br J Psychiatry 158:503–510, 1991

Lieberman J, Jody D, Geisler S, et al: Time course and biologic correlates of treatment response in first episode schizophrenia. Arch Gen Psychiatry 50:369–376, 1993

Lieberman JA, Koreen AR, Chakos M, et al: Factors influencing treatment response and outcome of first-episode schizophrenia: implications for understanding the pathophysiology of schizophrenia. J Clin Psychiatry 57 (suppl 9):5–9, 1996

Lieberman JA, Sheitman B, Chakos M, et al: The development of treatment resistance in patients with schizophrenia: a clinical and pathophysiologic perspective. J Clin Psychopharmacol 18 (2, suppl 1):20S–24S, 1998

Loebel AD, Lieberman JA, Alvir JMJ, et al: Duration of psychosis and outcome in first-episode schizophrenia. Am J Psychiatry 149:1183–1188, 1992

McEvoy JP, Hogarty GE, Steingard S: Optimal dose of neuroleptic in acute schizophrenia: a controlled study of the neuroleptic threshold and higher haloperidol dose. Arch Gen Psychiatry 48:739–745, 1991

Meltzer HY: An overview of the mechanism of action of clozapine. J Clin Psychiatry 55 (suppl B):47–52, 1994

Metzger E, Friedman R: Prolongation of the corrected QT and torsades de pointes cardiac arrhythmia associated with intravenous haloperidol in the medically ill. J Clin Psychopharmacol 13:128–132, 1993

Miller DD, Sharafuddin MJ, Kathol RG: A case of clozapine-induced neuroleptic malignant syndrome. J Clin Psychiatry 52:99–101, 1991

Nielsen H: Recombinant human granulocyte colony-stimulating factor (rhG-CSF; filgrastim) treatment of clozapine-induced agranulocytosis. J Intern Med 234:529–531, 1993

Oldham JM: Guideline Watch: Practice Guidelines for the Treatment of Patients With Borderline Personality Disorder. Arlington, VA, American Psychiatric Association, 2005

Oliver AP, Luchins DJ, Wyatt RJ: Neuroleptic-induced seizures: an in vitro technique for assessing relative risk. Arch Gen Psychiatry 39:206–209, 1982

Perry PJ, Miller DD, Arndt SV, et al: Clozapine and norclozapine plasma concentrations and clinical response of treatment-refractory schizophrenic patients. Am J Psychiatry 148:231–235, 1991

Petrie JL, Saha AR, McEvoy JP: Aripiprazole, a new atypical antipsychotic: overview of phase 2 results. Presentation at the 36th annual meeting of the American College of Neuropsychopharmacology, Waikoloa, HI, December 8–12, 1997

Physicians' Desk Reference, 51st Edition. Montvale, NJ, Medical Economics, 2001

Schooler NR, Keith SJ, Severe JB, et al: Relapse and rehospitalization during maintenance treatment of schizophrenia: the effects of dose reduction and family treatment. Arch Gen Psychiatry 54:453–463, 1997

Seroquel (package insert). Wilmington, DE, AstraZeneca, 2005

Silver JM, Yudofsky SC, Kogan M, et al: Elevation of thioridazine plasma levels by propranolol. Am J Psychiatry 143:1290–1292, 1986

Tollefson GD, Beasley CM Jr, Tamura RN: Blind, controlled long-term study of the comparative incidence of treatment-emergent tardive dyskinesia with olanzapine or haloperidol. Am J Psychiatry 154:1248–1254, 1997

Umbricht DS, Pollack S, Kane JM: Clozapine and weight gain. J Clin Psychiatry 55 (suppl B):157–160, 1994

Wetzel H, Anghelescu I, Szegedi A, et al: Pharmacokinetic interactions of clozapine with selective serotonin reuptake inhibitors: differential effects of fluvoxamine and paroxetine in a prospective study. J Clin Psychopharmacol 18:2–9, 1998

Zhang-Wong J, Zipursky RB, Beiser M, et al: Optimal haloperidol dosage in first-episode psychosis. Can J Psychiatry 44:164–167, 1999

5

MOOD STABILIZERS

Lithium, several (but not all) anticonvulsants, and most of the atypical antipsychotic medications are approved by the U.S. Food and Drug Administration (FDA) for the treatment of one or more phases of bipolar disorder. These medications are referred to as *mood stabilizers,* and they are the foundation of treatment for bipolar disorders. However, the skillful treatment of bipolar disorder requires not only the knowledge of how to prescribe one or more of these medications but also the understanding that some medications are preferred for one phase of the illness but not the other or for long-term use but not necessarily acute use. In this chapter, we first review the clinical use of lithium and the anticonvulsants that are definite or probable mood stabilizers. The general properties of atypical antipsychotics are reviewed in Chapter 4. In this chapter, we expand on the use of these compounds for the treatment of bipolar disorder. Discussion of the treatment of each phase of bipolar disorder concludes the chapter.

■ LITHIUM

Mechanism of Action

Lithium is a monovalent cation that inhibits several steps in phosphoinositide metabolism, as well as many second and third messengers, including G proteins and protein kinases. Recent evidence suggests that lithium ultimately stimulates neurite growth, regeneration, and neurogenesis, which is likely related to its therapeutic effect (Coyle et al. 2003; Kim et al. 2004).

Indications and Efficacy

Lithium has been proven effective for acute and prophylactic treatment of both manic and depressive episodes in patients with bipolar illness (American Psychiatric Association 2002). However, patients with rapid-cycling bipolar disorder (i.e., patients who experience four or more mood disorder episodes per year) have been reported to respond less well to lithium treatment (Dunner and Fieve 1974; Prien et al. 1984; Wehr et al. 1988). Lithium is also effective in preventing future depressive episodes in patients with recurrent unipolar depressive disorder (American Psychiatric Association 2002) and as an adjunct to antidepressant therapy in depressed patients whose illness is partially refractory to treatment with antidepressants alone (discussed in Chapter 2). Furthermore, lithium may be useful in maintaining remission of depressive disorders after electroconvulsive therapy (Coppen et al. 1981; Sackeim et al. 2001). Lithium also has been used effectively in some cases of aggression and behavioral dyscontrol.

Clinical Use

Lithium carbonate is completely absorbed by the gastrointestinal tract and reaches peak plasma levels in 1–2 hours. The elimination half-life is approximately 24 hours. Steady-state lithium levels are achieved in approximately 5 days. Therapeutic plasma levels range from 0.5 to 1.2 mEq/L. Lower plasma levels are associated with less troubling side effects, but levels of at least 0.8 mEq/L are often required in the treatment of acute manic episodes. Therefore, when intolerable side effects have not intervened, treatment of acute mania with lithium should not be considered a failure until plasma levels of 1.0–1.2 mEq/L have been reached and have been maintained for 2 weeks. As discussed at the end of this chapter (see "Treatment of Mania or Mixed Episodes"), more severely ill patients may require combination treatment.

Serum concentrations required for prophylaxis are not as well determined. The only controlled trial of patients randomly assigned to a low lithium level (0.4–0.6 mEq/L) compared with a standard-dose lithium group (0.8–1.0 mEq/L) found fewer recurrences in the standard-dose group (Gelenberg et al. 1989); however, a reanalysis of these data indicated that an abrupt decrease in serum lithium level may be a more powerful predictor of recurrence of bipolar disorder than is the absolute assignment to a low or a standard dose of lithium (Perlis et al. 2002). Although the prophylactic efficacy of lithium levels between 0.6 and 0.8 mEq/L has not been studied in a controlled clinical trial, clinical experience suggests that this range is commonly used to balance efficacy and dose-dependent side effects.

Because lithium has a serum half-life of approximately 24 hours, it may be administered as a single daily dose. Evening dosing is preferred because some side effects, such as tremor, are associated with peak blood levels. Lithium levels should be determined 12 hours after the last lithium dose. After therapeutic lithium levels have been established, levels should be measured every month for the first 3 months and every 3 months thereafter. In patients who have remained stable and who are aware of early signs of both relapse and lithium toxicity, lithium levels may be measured less frequently. In addition, serum urea nitrogen and creatinine levels should be measured before lithium therapy has commenced and every 3–6 months during therapy, with more frequent testing if there are specific complaints or signs of renal dysfunction.

Contraindications and Pretreatment Medical Evaluation

Lithium should not be administered to patients with fluctuating or unstable renal function. Because lithium may affect functioning of the cardiac sinus node, patients with sinus node dysfunction (e.g., sick sinus syndrome) should not receive lithium. Although lithium also has acute and chronic effects on the thyroid, patients with hypothyroidism may receive lithium if the thyroid disease is adequately treated and monitored. Laboratory tests that should be performed before initiation of lithium are listed in Table 5–1.

The risk of Ebstein's anomaly in infants exposed to lithium in utero is 0.1%–0.7% (Edmonds and Oakley 1990; Jacobson et al. 1992; Kallen and Tandberg 1983; Zalzstein et al. 1990), compared with 0.01% in the general population. The overall risk of major con-

TABLE 5-1. Characteristics of mood stabilizers[a]

	Lithium	Valproate	Carbamazepine	Lamotrigine
Available preparations	Lithium carbonate (Eskalith, Lithonate, Lithotabs; 150, 300, 600-mg tablets, capsules) Lithium citrate liquid (8 mEq/5 mL) Extended-release lithium (Eskalith CR, 450 mg; Lithobid, 300 mg)	Divalproex sodium (Depakote, 125-, 250-, 500-mg tablets; 125-mg sprinkle capsules) Valproate sodium injection (Depacon) Valproic acid (Depakene, 250-mg capsules; 250 mg/5 mL syrup) Extended-release divalproex sodium (Depakote ER, 250, 500 mg)	Carbamazepine (Tegretol; 100-mg chewable tablets; 200-mg tablets) Extended-release carbamazepine capsules (Equetro, 100, 200, 300 mg; Carbatrol, 200, 300 mg) Carbamazepine suspension (100 mg/5 mL) Extended-release carbamazepine tablets (Tegretol XR, 100, 200, 400 mg)	Lamotrigine (Lamictal, 25-, 100-, 150-, 200-mg tablets; Lamictal CD [chewable dispersible], 2-, 5-, 25-mg tablets)

TABLE 5-1. Characteristics of mood stabilizers[a] (continued)

	Lithium	Valproate	Carbamazepine	Lamotrigine
Half-life (hours)	24	96	Initially, 25–65; decreases to 12–17 because of autoinduction	25–33[b]
Starting dosage	300 mg twice daily	250 mg three times a day or 20 mg/kg[c]	Tablets/capsules: 200 mg twice daily[d]; suspension: 100 mg four times a day	25 mg/day[b]
Blood level	0.8–1.2 mEq/L	45–125 μg/mL	Not helpful; monitor for signs/ symptoms of toxicity	Not monitored; target dose of lamotrigine is 200 mg/day
Metabolism	Renal	Hepatic	Hepatic	Hepatic
Contraindications[e]	Unstable renal function	Hepatic dysfunction	Hepatic dysfunction, bone marrow suppression	Previous hypersensitivity to lamotrigine

TABLE 5–1. **Characteristics of mood stabilizers[a] (continued)**

	Lithium	Valproate	Carbamazepine	Lamotrigine
Key side effects, risks, and features	Nephrogenic diabetes insipidus	Titration or loading dose strategies	Cytochrome P450 inducer (oral contraceptive failure)	Rash risk in 5%–10%
	Reversible hypothyroidism	Rare hepatotoxicity		Rarely, life-threatening rash (including Stevens-Johnson syndrome)
	Tremor	Rare pancreatitis	Autoinduction	
	Benign leukocytosis	Polycystic ovarian syndrome	Rare blood cell dyscrasias: aplastic anemia, agranulocytosis	Risk minimized by low starting dose and slow titration
	Weight gain	Weight gain		
	Narrow therapeutic index	Tremor	Hepatotoxicity	Metabolism inhibited by valproate
	Potentially fatal toxicity	Alopecia	Rash risk, including Stevens-Johnson syndrome	Metabolism induced by carbamazepine
	Risk of Ebstein's anomaly with first-trimester exposure	Rare blood cell dyscrasias	Risk for SIADH	
		Risk of neural tube defects with first-trimester exposure	Teratogenicity risk: neural tube defects, craniofacial defects	

TABLE 5–1. Characteristics of mood stabilizers[a] *(continued)*

	Lithium	Valproate	Carbamazepine	Lamotrigine
Pretreatment laboratory evaluation	Chem 20,[f] CBC, TSH level determination, ECG (if patient is 40 years or older or has cardiac disease), pregnancy test	AST and ALT level determinations, pregnancy test	AST, ALT, CBC, sodium level, pregnancy test	None; might consider a pregnancy test

Note. SIADH=syndrome of inappropriate secretion of antidiuretic hormone; CBC=complete blood count; TSH=thyroid-stimulating hormone; ECG=electrocardiogram; AST=aspartate aminotransaminase; ALT=alanine aminotransaminase.

[a]The atypical antipsychotics are presented in Chapter 4.

[b]Approximately doubles with valproate and decreases by approximately half with carbamazepine/primidone/phenytoin/phenobarbital/rifampin; therefore, initial doses may vary depending on concomitant medications.

[c]Increase dose by 10%–20% when converting from valproate, divalproex, or valproic acid to the extended-release (ER) formulation of divalproex sodium.

[d]100 mg twice daily if given in combination with a neuroleptic or lithium.

[e]Lithium, valproate, and carbamazepine should be avoided in pregnancy, if possible; see text for discussion.

[f]Especially serum urea nitrogen, creatinine, sodium, and calcium levels.

genital anomalies associated with lithium exposure is 4%–12%, compared with 2%–4% in comparison groups (Cohen et al. 1994). The increased risk of malformations must be weighed against the risk of harm to both mother and fetus if lithium discontinuation results in a manic relapse.

Risks, Side Effects, and Their Management

Renal Effects

In the absence of toxicity, the effects of lithium on the kidneys are largely reversible after discontinuation of the drug. Lithium inhibits vasopressin, leading to impairment in renal concentrating ability. This condition, called *nephrogenic diabetes insipidus,* results in polyuria in up to 60% of patients taking lithium. Diuretics may be used in the treatment of lithium-induced nephrogenic diabetes insipidus. By causing sodium depletion, diuretics ultimately create in the kidneys a compensatory conservation of sodium. The osmotic effect of this sodium conservation constrains the kidneys' ability to dilute urine, thereby alleviating the polyuria. However, the addition of thiazide diuretics in a patient taking lithium may result in increased lithium levels to the toxic range. Amiloride apparently acts by blocking absorption of lithium in the renal tubules, where the lithium would otherwise interfere with the action of vasopressin. For lithium-induced nephrogenic diabetes insipidus, amiloride is prescribed at a dosage of 5 mg twice daily, with an increase to 10 mg twice daily if necessary.

Permanent morphological changes in renal structure have been reported in patients who have experienced lithium toxicity (Markowitz et al. 2000). Case reports of irreversible renal failure as a result of chronic, nontoxic lithium therapy are extremely rare and typically follow 10 or more years of treatment, during which time the patient's serum creatinine levels have gradually increased (e.g., to 2.0 mg/100 mL; Gitlin 1993). To minimize the risk of renal complications, which are rare but potentially serious, we recommend frequent patient education about the risks of toxicity and factors that might make toxicity more likely, such as drug interactions or dehydration. A nephrology consultation is warranted if routine laboratory monitoring detects a pattern of rising serum creatinine levels. This pattern is typically observed over many years.

Thyroid Dysfunction

Reversible hypothyroidism may occur in as many as 20% of the patients receiving lithium (Lindstedt et al. 1977; Myers et al. 1985). Lithium-induced hypothyroidism occurs more frequently in women. Thyroid function should be evaluated every 6–12 months during lithium treatment or if symptoms develop that might be attributable to thyroid dysfunction, including depression or rapid cycling.

Parathyroid Dysfunction

Clinically significant effects of hypercalcemia associated with lithium therapy have been reported, including back pain, kyphoscoliosis, osteoporosis, hypertension, cardiomegaly, and impaired renal function. Although they are rare, symptoms of hyperparathyroidism may be misdiagnosed as lithium toxicity or the effects of the underlying mood disorder. When signs or symptoms that might be related to hyperparathyroidism develop, serum calcium ion levels should be checked, and if they are abnormal, parathyroid hormone levels should be measured and an endocrinologist consulted.

Neurotoxicity

A fine resting tremor is a common side effect. β-Adrenergic-blocking drugs, such as propranolol (<80 mg/day in divided doses), are effective in treating this tremor. Subjective memory impairment commonly occurs and is among the most frequent reasons for noncompliance (Goodwin and Jamison 1990).

Cardiac Effects

Benign flattening of the T wave on the electrocardiogram occurs in 20%–30% of patients taking lithium (Bucht et al. 1984). In addition, lithium may suppress the function of the sinus node and result in sinoatrial block. An electrocardiogram should be obtained before treatment with lithium is started in patients older than 40 years or in those with a history or symptoms of cardiac disease.

Weight Gain

Weight gain is a frequent side effect of lithium treatment.

Dermatological Effects

Dermatological reactions to lithium include acne, follicular eruptions, and psoriasis. Hair loss and thinning also have been reported. Except for cases of exacerbation of psoriasis, these reactions are usually benign and may not warrant discontinuation of lithium treatment. Lithium-induced acne responds to topical treatment with retinoid acid, such as tretinoin (Retin-A).

Gastrointestinal Symptoms

Nausea and diarrhea are common early side effects. Gastrointestinal symptoms may improve with dose reduction or with ingestion of lithium at meals. Slow-release formulations are more often associated with nausea, whereas sustained-release preparations are more commonly associated with diarrhea.

Hematological Effects

The hematological change most frequently detected in patients taking lithium is leukocytosis (approximately 15,000 white blood cells/mm^3). This change is generally benign and reversible.

Overdose and Toxicity

Given the narrow margin between therapeutic and toxic plasma lithium levels, the physician must emphasize the prevention of lithium toxicity through adequate salt and water intake, especially during hot weather and exercise. Toxic lithium levels can cause severe neurotoxic reactions, with symptoms such as dysarthria, ataxia, and intention tremor. The signs and symptoms of lithium toxicity may be divided into those that usually occur at lithium levels between 1.5 and 2.0 mEq/L, those that occur at lithium levels greater than 2.0 mEq/L but not more than 2.5 mEq/L, and those that occur at levels greater than 2.5 mEq/L (Table 5–2), although some patients may experience clinical toxicity when lithium levels are in the standard therapeutic range. The recommended management of lithium toxicity is outlined in Table 5–3.

Drug Interactions

Given the narrow therapeutic range of lithium doses, knowledge of the interactions between lithium and other drugs is of paramount importance. Because the kidneys excrete lithium, any medication that alters renal function can affect lithium levels. Thiazide diuretics reduce lithium clearance and hence may increase lithium levels. Loop diuretics (e.g., furosemide) do not have this effect. Nonsteroidal anti-inflammatory drugs also may increase lithium levels by decreasing clearance. It is particularly important to inform patients of this effect because these medications are commonly self prescribed. Other medications that may increase lithium levels include angiotensin-converting enzyme inhibitors and cyclooxygenase-2 inhibitors (e.g., celecoxib, rofecoxib). Drugs that may decrease lithium levels include theophylline and aminophylline. Lithium may potentiate the effects of succinylcholine-like muscle relaxants.

■ VALPROATE

Divalproex sodium was approved by the FDA for the treatment of mania and is commonly used for all phases of bipolar disorder, as well as mood instability due to other causes.

Mechanism of Action

Although many mechanisms have been proposed, the basis for the mood-stabilizing effects of valproate is most likely concordant with

TABLE 5–2.	Signs and symptoms of lithium toxicity

Mild to moderate intoxication (lithium level=1.5–2.0 mEq/L)

Gastrointestinal symptoms
Vomiting
Abdominal pain
Dryness of mouth

Neurological symptoms
Ataxia
Dizziness
Slurred speech
Nystagmus
Lethargy or excitement
Muscle weakness

Moderate to severe intoxication (lithium level=2.1–2.5 mEq/L)

Gastrointestinal symptoms
Anorexia
Persistent nausea and vomiting

Neurological symptoms
Blurred vision
Muscle fasciculations
Clonic limb movements
Hyperactive deep tendon reflexes
Choreoathetoid movements
Convulsions
Delirium
Syncope
Electroencephalographic changes
Stupor
Coma
Circulatory failure (decreased blood pressure, cardiac arrhythmias, conduction abnormalities)

Severe intoxication (lithium level>2.5 mEq/L)
Generalized convulsions
Oliguria and renal failure
Death

TABLE 5–3.   **Management of lithium toxicity**

---

1. The patient should immediately contact his or her personal physician or go to a hospital emergency department.

2. Lithium should be discontinued, and the patient should ingest fluids if possible.

3. A physical examination (including checking of vital signs) and a neurological examination (including a complete, formal mental status examination) should be performed.

4. As soon as possible, lithium and serum electrolyte levels should be measured, renal function tests performed, and an electrocardiogram obtained.

5. In cases of significant acute ingestion, residual gastric contents should be removed by induction of emesis, gastric lavage, and absorption with activated charcoal.[a]

6. Vigorous hydration and maintenance of electrolyte balance are essential.

7. In a patient with a serum lithium level greater than 4.0 mEq/L or with serious manifestations of lithium toxicity, hemodialysis should be initiated.[a]

8. Repeat dialysis may be required every 6–10 hours, until the lithium level is within nontoxic range and the patient has no signs or symptoms of lithium toxicity.

---

[a]Information from Goldfrank et al. 1986.

lithium's mechanism of action—specifically, attenuation of the activity of protein kinase C and other steps in the signal transduction pathway, leading to neuronal adaptation and changes in gene expression (Chen et al. 1994; Manji et al. 1996), including neurotrophic effects (Coyle and Duman 2003).

Clinical Use

Before starting treatment with valproate, patients should be told that they might experience nausea, sedation, and a fine hand tremor. These effects are often transient, but in some patients they persist.

Several valproate preparations are available in the United States, including valproic acid, sodium valproate, divalproex sodium, and an extended-release preparation of divalproex sodium. Divalproex sodium is a dimer of sodium valproate and valproic acid with an enteric coating, and it is much better tolerated than other oral valproate preparations. An intravenous preparation also has become available, but it has not been well studied in patients with psychiatric disorders. The half-life of valproate is 9–16 hours.

Valproate therapy may be initiated gradually, with subsequent dose titration; alternatively, a more rapid, "loading" strategy may be used. Most commonly, treatment with valproate is initiated at a dosage of 250 mg three times a day, with subsequent increases of 250 mg every 3 days. Most patients require a daily dose of 1,250–2,000 mg. Although valproate has a relatively short half-life, moderate doses may be given once a day at bedtime to reduce daytime sedation; such dosing often does not compromise clinical efficacy. This strategy should not be used when the drug is being used to treat seizure disorders, for which more constant serum levels are required.

When rapid stabilization is required, valproate treatment can be initiated at a dose of 20 mg per kilogram of body weight (Keck et al. 1993). Some patients require relatively high doses of valproate, sometimes greater than 4,000 mg/day, to achieve a sufficient plasma level and clinical response, and some patients do not respond until plasma valproate levels are greater than 100 μg/mL. As with other psychotropic medications, dosing should be based on the balance between clinical response and side effects rather than on absolute blood level. However, plasma levels of 45–100 μg/mL are recommended for the treatment of acute mania (Bowden et al. 1996). Patients with less severe disorders, such as bipolar II disorder or cyclothymia, often respond at lower doses and blood levels (Jacobsen 1993). Blood levels for other phases of bipolar disorder, such as bipolar depression, or for other indications, such as aggression, have not been established. The extended-release preparation of divalproex sodium has 80%–90% of the bioavailability of the initial divalproex sodium, so doses may need to be slightly higher when this preparation is used.

Contraindications

Valproate is relatively contraindicated in patients with hepatitis or liver disease; in such patients, it may be used only as a last resort and with the approval and continuous involvement of a gastroenterologist. Valproate has been linked to spina bifida and other neural tube defects in the offspring of patients exposed to this medication in the first trimester of pregnancy (Lammer et al. 1987; Robert and Guibaud 1982). The first trimester is the time of highest risk because that is when the neural tube is forming. The risks of continuing valproate therapy during pregnancy must be balanced against the risk of relapse. Abrupt discontinuation of medication in a woman with severe illness who is otherwise stable while taking valproate in the second or third trimester of pregnancy may be more harmful than helpful

Risks, Side Effects, and Their Management

Hepatic Toxicity

Although it is estimated that 1 in 118,000 patients dies from non-dose-related hepatic failure, no cases have occurred in patients older than 10 years who were receiving valproate monotherapy. Nonetheless, baseline liver function tests are indicated. If baseline test results are normal, monitoring for clinical signs of hepatotoxicity is more important than routine monitoring of liver enzyme levels, which has little predictive value and may be less effective than clinical monitoring (Pellock and Willmore 1991).

Transient, mild increases in liver enzyme levels, up to three times the upper limit of normal, do not necessitate discontinuation of valproate. Although γ-glutamyltransferase levels are often checked by clinicians, these levels are often increased, without clinical significance, in patients receiving valproate and carbamazepine (Dean and Penry 1992). Likewise, plasma ammonia levels are often increased transiently during valproate treatment, but this finding does not necessitate interruption of treatment (Jaeken et al. 1980). Increases in transaminase levels are often dose dependent. If no suitable alternative treatment is available, dose reduction (with careful monitoring) may be attempted.

Hematological Effects

Valproate has been associated with changes in platelet counts, but clinically significant thrombocytopenia has rarely been documented. Coagulation defects also have been reported. Overall, the risk of inducing a coagulation disturbance in an otherwise healthy adult is extremely low. However, in patients in whom anticoagulation is strictly contraindicated and in patients who are already receiving anticoagulation therapy, monitoring of the coagulation profile is required at baseline, after 1 month of therapy, and then at least every 3 months.

Gastrointestinal Symptoms

Indigestion, heartburn, and nausea are common side effects of valproate therapy. Use of the divalproex sodium preparation will help mitigate these effects. Patients may also be encouraged to take their doses with food. The symptomatic use of histamine H_2 blockers, such as famotidine, is sometimes warranted. In most cases, however, dyspepsia is transient and not severe. Pancreatitis is a rare occurrence in patients receiving relatively high doses of valproate. If vomiting and severe abdominal pain develop during valproate therapy, serum amylase levels should be determined immediately.

Weight Gain

Weight gain is a common side effect of valproate treatment. Isojarvi et al. (1996) reported significant weight gain with associated hyperinsulinemia in approximately 50% of a cohort of women taking valproate. This side effect does not appear to be dose dependent. Diet and exercise should be recommended early in treatment.

Neurological Effects

One of the most common side effects of valproate therapy is benign essential tremor. Drowsiness is another common side effect, but tolerance often develops once a steady-state level of the drug is reached. In addition, once-daily dosing at bedtime often achieves symptomatic remission with less daytime sedation.

Alopecia

Both transient and persistent hair loss have been associated with valproate use. Patients with valproate-induced alopecia may benefit from zinc supplementation, at a dose of 22.5 mg/day (Hurd et al. 1984).

Polycystic Ovarian Syndrome

Polycystic ovarian syndrome is characterized by menstrual irregularity, hyperandrogenism, and the exclusion of other etiologies. Isojarvi et al. (1993) reported an association between polycystic ovarian syndrome and valproate in women receiving long-term valproate treatment for epilepsy, especially those who were younger than 20. Until recently, it was not clear that a similar phenomenon occurred in women with bipolar disorder. However, recent data from the Systematic Treatment Enhancement Program for Bipolar Disorders indicated that women taking valproate alone or in combination had an 11% rate of polycystic ovaries or hyperandrogenism, compared with 1.4% of women with bipolar disorder who were not taking valproate (Joffe et al., in press). Given these data, clinicians should document menstrual irregularities and observe for signs of hyperandrogenism, such as hirsutism.

Overdose

Valproate overdose results in increasing sedation, confusion, and ultimately, coma. The patient may also manifest hyperreflexia or hyporeflexia, seizures, respiratory suppression, and supraventricular tachycardia. Treatment should include gastric lavage, electrocardiographic monitoring, treatment of emergent seizures, and respiratory support.

Drug Interactions

Because valproate may inhibit hepatic enzymes, there is the potential for increases in levels of other medications. Valproate is also highly bound to plasma proteins and may displace other highly bound drugs from protein-binding sites. Therefore, coadministered drugs that are either highly protein bound or reliant on hepatic metabolism may require dose adjustment. Drugs that may increase valproate levels include cimetidine, macrolide antibiotics (e.g., erythromycin), and felbamate.

Valproate may increase concentrations of phenobarbital, ethosuximide, and the active 10,11-epoxide metabolite of carbamazepine, increasing the risk of toxicity. Valproate may also raise lamotrigine levels, increasing the risk of rash.

Valproate metabolism may be induced by other anticonvulsants, including carbamazepine, phenytoin, primidone, and phenobarbital, resulting in an increased total clearance of valproate and perhaps decreased efficacy.

■ CARBAMAZEPINE

Carbamazepine is effective in both acute and prophylactic treatment of mania (Weisler et al. 2005). An extended-release formulation of carbamazepine, available since 1997 for treatment of epilepsy, was approved in 2004 under the brand name Equetro. Extended-release preparations are preferred because simplified dosage schedules facilitate patient adherence. Other extended-release carbamazepine preparations include Tegretol XR and Carbatrol, although neither has been specifically indicated for the treatment of bipolar disorder. The longer-acting preparations are also of benefit because they tend to have fewer gastrointestinal side effects.

Clinical Use

Carbamazepine should be initiated at a dosage of 200 mg twice a day, with increases in increments of 200 mg/day every 3–5 days. Cited plasma levels of 8–12 μg/mL are based on clinical use in patients with seizure disorders and do not correlate with clinical response in patients with psychiatric disorders. We recommend dose titration to achieve clinical response and minimize side effects rather than focusing on a particular dose or blood level. During the titration phase, patients may be particularly prone to side effects such as sedation, dizziness, and ataxia; if these occur, titration should be more gradual (the dosage might be 100 mg twice a day, for example). Because carbamazepine induces its own metabolism (autoinduction), dose adjustments may be required for weeks or months after initiation of treatment to maintain therapeutic plasma levels.

Contraindications

Because of the potential for hematological and hepatic toxicity, carbamazepine should not be administered to patients with liver disease or thrombocytopenia or to those at risk for agranulocytosis. For this reason, carbamazepine is strictly contraindicated in patients receiving clozapine. Because of reports of teratogenicity, including increased risks of spina bifida (Rosa 1991), microcephaly (Bertollini et al. 1987), and craniofacial defects (Jones et al. 1989), carbamazepine is relatively contraindicated in pregnant women. Pretreatment evaluation should include a complete blood count and determination of alanine aminotransferase (ALT) and aspartate aminotransferase (AST) levels.

Risks, Side Effects, and Their Management

Hematological Effects

The most serious toxic hematological side effects of carbamazepine are agranulocytosis and aplastic anemia, which can be fatal. Whereas carbamazepine-induced agranulocytosis or aplastic anemia are extremely rare, other hematological effects, such as leukopenia (total white blood cell count<3,000 cells/mm^3), thrombocytopenia, and mild anemia may occur more frequently. Although it is important to assess hematological function and risk factors before initiating treatment, there appears to be no benefit to ongoing monitoring in the absence of clinical indicators. When carbamazepine-induced agranulocytosis occurs, the onset is rapid. Thus, a normal complete blood count one day does not mean that agranulocytosis will not develop the next day. Therefore, it is more important to educate the patient to early signs and symptoms of agranulocytosis and thrombocytopenia and to tell the patient to inform the psychiatrist immediately if these signs and symptoms develop.

Hepatic Toxicity

Carbamazepine therapy is occasionally associated with hepatic toxicity, usually a hypersensitivity hepatitis that appears after a latency period of several weeks and involves increases in ALT, AST, and lactate dehydrogenase levels. Cholestasis is also possible, with increases in bilirubin and alkaline phosphatase concentrations. Mild, transient increases in transaminase levels generally do not necessitate discontinuation of carbamazepine. If ALT or AST levels increase more than three times the upper limit of normal, carbamazepine should be discontinued.

Dermatological Effects

An exanthematous rash is one of the more common side effects of carbamazepine, occurring in 3%–17% of patients. This reaction typically begins within 2–20 weeks after the start of treatment. Carbamazepine is generally discontinued if a rash develops because of the risk of progression to an exfoliative dermatitis or Stevens-Johnson syndrome, a severe bullous form of erythema multiforme.

Endocrine Disorders

The syndrome of inappropriate antidiuretic hormone secretion, with resultant hyponatremia, may be induced by carbamazepine treatment. Alcoholic patients may be at greater risk for hyponatremia.

Weight Gain

Weight gain does not appear to be a side effect of carbamazepine therapy.

Gastrointestinal Symptoms

Nausea and occasional vomiting are common side effects of carbamazepine.

Neurological Effects

Patients may develop dizziness, drowsiness, or ataxia. These symptoms often occur at therapeutic plasma levels, especially in the early phases of treatment, and in such cases, the dose should be reduced and a slower titration schedule implemented.

Overdose

Carbamazepine overdose first leads to neuromuscular disturbances, such as nystagmus, myoclonus, and hyperreflexia, with later progression to seizures and coma. Cardiac conduction changes are possible. Nausea, vomiting, and urinary retention also may occur. Treatment should include induction of vomiting, gastric lavage, and supportive care. After a serious overdose, blood pressure and respiratory and kidney function should be monitored for several days.

Drug Interactions

Carbamazepine induces hepatic cytochrome P450 (CYP) enzymes, which may reduce levels of other medications. Through the mechanism of hepatic enzyme induction, carbamazepine therapy can lead to oral contraceptive failure; therefore, women should be advised to consider alternative forms of birth control while taking carbamazepine. Similarly, use of medications or substances that inhibit CYP 3A3/4 (discussed in Chapter 1) may result in significant increases in plasma carbamazepine levels.

■ LAMOTRIGINE

Lamotrigine is an anticonvulsant medication that decreases sustained high-frequency repetitive firing of the voltage-dependent sodium channel, which may then decrease glutamate release (Leach et al. 1991; Macdonald and Kelly 1995). Lamotrigine is approved by the FDA for the prevention of mania and depression in patients with bipolar disorder. Two separate randomized controlled trials showed a greater time to intervention for any mood episode for both lamotrigine and lithium compared with placebo (Bowden et al. 2003; Calabrese et al. 2003). Of interest, in these trials, lamotrigine was predominantly effective against the prevention of depression, and lithium was predominantly effective against the prevention of mania.

Unlike most other medications used to treat bipolar disorder, lamotrigine is not effective in the acute treatment of mania. Lamotrigine has shown efficacy in a double-blind, placebo-controlled trial for the treatment of bipolar depression (Calabrese et al. 1999), although this result has not yet been confirmed, and is frequently used for the acute and longer-term control of the depressed phase of bipolar disorder (American Psychiatric Association 2002; Marangell et al. 2004). In addition, a 6-month study involving patients with rapid-cycling bipolar disorder found that lamotrigine monotherapy was more effective than placebo in preventing relapse, especially in patients with bipolar II disorder (Calabrese et al. 2000).

Clinical Use

Lamotrigine requires slow dose titration to minimize the risk of skin rash. Lamotrigine treatment is usually initiated at 25 mg once a day. Because the risk of a serious rash increases with rapid titration, it is essential to follow the recommended titration schedule, regardless of the severity of illness. After 2 weeks, the dose is increased to 50 mg/day for another 2 weeks. At week 5, the dose can be increased to 100 mg/day and at week 6 to 200 mg/day. In patients who are taking valproate or other medications that decrease the clearance of lamotrigine, the dosing schedule and target dose are halved. Conversely, the titration schedule and dose are increased in those taking carbamazepine. In the absence of carbamazepine or other enzyme inducers, doses higher than 200 mg are typically not recommended in the treatment of bipolar disorder. Lamotrigine is mildly activating in many patients. Therefore, we recommend morning administration of the medication, especially if the patient complains of insomnia.

Risks, Side Effects, and Their Management

Lamotrigine is well tolerated and is not associated with hepatotoxicity, weight gain, or significant sedation. Common early side effects include headache, dizziness, gastrointestinal distress, and blurred or double vision. The most serious potential side effect is rash (described in the following subsection).

Rash

A maculopapular rash develops in 5%–10% of patients taking lamotrigine, usually in the first 8 weeks of treatment. Serious rashes requiring hospitalization and discontinuation of treatment may occur. The incidence of these rashes, which have included Stevens-Johnson syndrome, is approximately 0.08% (0.8 per 1,000). Stevens-Johnson syndrome is potentially fatal. Patients must be advised of this risk and of the necessity to call the office at once if they develop a rash. Development of a rash with concomitant systemic symptoms is a particularly ominous sign, and the patient should be evaluated immediately.

The risk of a rash is minimized by following the prescribed titration schedule, including using a slower titration for patients who are also taking valproate. In addition, Ketter and colleagues (2005) reported a decreased incidence of treatment-emergent rash by advising patients who are starting lamotrigine to avoid other new medicines and new foods, cosmetics, conditioners, deodorants, detergents, and fabric softeners, as well as sunburn and exposure to poison ivy and poison oak. Ketter et al. further recommend not starting lamotrigine within 2 weeks of a rash, viral syndrome, or vaccination.

Drug Interactions

Oral contraceptives can result in decreases in lamotrigine concentrations. In women taking lamotrigine and oral contraceptives, lamotrigine should be carefully increased to compensate for this pharmacokinetic interaction. Conversely, when oral contraceptives are discontinued, the clinician should decrease the lamotrigine dose. Lamotrigine does not affect the availability of oral contraceptives. Many other anticonvulsants interact with lamotrigine. Most germane to bipolar disorders, valproate will increase lamotrigine levels, and carbamazepine will decrease lamotrigine levels.

■ OXCARBAZEPINE

Oxcarbazepine is a keto derivative of carbamazepine but offers several advantages over carbamazepine. Oxcarbazepine does not require blood cell count, hepatic, or serum drug level monitoring. It causes less cytochrome P450 enzyme induction than does carbamazepine (but may decrease effectiveness of oral contraceptives containing ethinyl estradiol and levonorgestrel). As opposed to carbamazepine, oxcarbazepine does not induce its own metabolism. These properties, combined with its similarity to carbamazepine, led many clinicians to use this medication for the treatment of bipolar disorder. Randomized controlled trials suggested efficacy in the treatment of acute mania compared with lithium and haloperidol, but these trials were quite small and did not include a placebo control (Emrich 1990).

Oxcarbazepine is typically started at a dosage of 150 mg twice a day and titrated by 300 mg/day at weekly intervals. Therapeutic dosages are in the range of 450 mg twice a day to 1,200 mg twice a day. The conversion from carbamazepine to oxcarbazepine is approximately 1 to 1.5. Oxcarbazepine has a higher risk of hyponatremia than does carbamazepine. Serum sodium should be monitored in patients at risk for hyponatremia, such as the elderly or patients who are also taking diuretics. Stevens-Johnson syndrome and toxic epidermal necrolysis may occur between 3 and 10 times more frequently in oxcarbazepine-treated patients than in the general population. Median time from starting treatment to the development of these serious reactions is 19 days.

■ OTHER ANTICONVULSANTS

Virtually all anticonvulsants are or have been of interest for the treatment of bipolar disorder. However, the importance of controlled data cannot be understated. For example, gabapentin, an anticonvulsant that initially received much attention as a potential mood stabilizer, was compared with placebo and did not appear to stabilize mood (Frye et al. 2000; Pande et al. 2000). Similar negative results were seen with topiramate in placebo-controlled trials for the treatment of mania. Although these medications might be useful adjuncts in some patients, given the currently expanded pharmacopoeia of medications with positive controlled trial data in bipolar disorder, we do not recommend the primary use of agents that have only case reports as an evidence base or controlled studies with predominantly negative results.

■ ATYPICAL ANTIPSYCHOTICS

The clinical use and side effects of the atypical antipsychotics are reviewed in Chapter 4. All of the atypical antipsychotic medications, except clozapine, are approved by the FDA for the treatment of acute mania. Clinicians must remember that the efficacy of the atypical antipsychotics in the treatment of mania is independent of the presence or absence of psychotic symptoms. Indeed, across randomized controlled clinical trials, atypical antipsychotics have shown efficacy in treating the core symptoms of mania, such as elevated mood, increased motor activity, and increased speech. General dosing guidelines for acute mania are shown in Table 5–4. It is common clinical practice to use lower starting dosages for patients who are less ill, particularly those patients receiving treatment in outpatient settings who may discontinue treatment in the face of early side effects, but this practice has not been studied in randomized controlled trials. At present, only two of the atypical antipsychotics—olanzapine and aripiprazole—have been approved by the FDA as maintenance-phase treatments for bipolar disorder, although studies are under way with the other agents. The use of these agents for the depressed phase of bipolar disorder is an area of active clinical investigation. Clozapine has not received FDA approval for use in bipolar disorder, but it is a valuable option for patients whose symptoms are otherwise resistant to treatment (Suppes et al. 1999). Conventional antipsychotics should be avoided because they are associated with more extrapyramidal side effects and a greater risk of tardive dyskinesia compared with atypical antipsychotics.

Olanzapine-Fluoxetine Combination

The olanzapine-fluoxetine combination is currently the only medication approved by the FDA specifically for the treatment of depression in patients with bipolar disorder. This indication was based on data from a double-blind, randomized study in which the combination was superior to both olanzapine monotherapy and placebo (Tohen et al. 2003). Treatment-emergent mania or hypomania did not occur more frequently in the olanzapine-fluoxetine combination group than in the placebo group during the acute trial.

Clinical Use

The olanzapine-fluoxetine combination is available in four dosing preparations (6 mg/25 mg, 12 mg/25 mg, 6 mg/50 mg, 12 mg/50 mg) that allow clinicians to tailor treatment individually to provide greater or lesser amounts of each medication component. The typical starting dose for most patients is 6 mg/25 mg. Common side effects include somnolence, weight gain, increased appetite, asthenia, peripheral edema, and tremor. As one might expect, warnings and precautions that apply to either fluoxetine or olanzapine also apply to this combination treatment. For example, concomitant use of monoamine oxidase inhibitors is contraindicated given the fluoxetine component. Similarly, warnings and precautions regarding the potential association between olanzapine and hyperglycemia also apply. Additionally, clinicians should be aware of the potential drug-drug interactions that apply to either fluoxetine or olanzapine alone, such as the potential for clinically relevant CYP 2D6 isoenzyme inhibition by the fluoxetine component.

TABLE 5–4. Summary of atypical antipsychotic dosing in acute mania

Drug	Key features	Dosing in acute mania (mg/day)[a]		
		Starting dose	Dose titration	Target dose
Olanzapine	Moderate weight gain, somnolence	10–15	5 mg/day increments	5–20
Risperidone	Mild weight gain, EPS at high doses	2–3	1 mg/day increments	1–6
Aripiprazole	Akathisia, typically weight neutral	15–30	15 mg increments	30
Quetiapine	Sedation, mild weight gain, orthostatic hypotension	100	50–100 mg/day increments	600
Ziprasidone	Risk of prolonged QTc; typically weight neutral	80 (divided twice daily)	40–80 mg/day increments	120–160

Note.   EPS=extrapyramidal symptoms; QTc=corrected QT interval on the electrocardiogram.
[a]Lower dosages and slower titrations are indicated for the elderly.

■ TREATMENT OF MANIA OR MIXED EPISODES

The first step in the treatment of mania is to initiate treatment with one or two mood stabilizers with acute antimanic properties (American Psychiatric Association 2002). Lithium, valproate, carbamazepine, olanzapine, risperidone, aripiprazole, quetiapine, and ziprasidone are all indicated as single agents for the treatment of mania. Olanzapine and ziprasidone are also available in an injectable preparation. In patients who are severely ill or who have manic or mixed states with psychotic features, the American Psychiatric Association (2002) practice guideline recommends initial treatment with the combination of lithium or valproate and an atypical antipsychotic. This recommendation is based on several randomized controlled trials that have found more consistent antimanic effects and/or a faster onset of action with combination treatment compared with monotherapy (Tohen et al. 2000). For less severely ill patients, monotherapy is begun first if the patient is not taking a mood stabilizer; if the patient is already taking a mood stabilizer, the dose of the current medication should be optimized. Starting doses and rapidity of titration depend on balancing the clinical need for rapid control of symptoms, which dictates faster titration, with the improved tolerability of slower dose escalations. As with other classes of medication, the choice of medications is based on prior response, comorbid illnesses, and the varying side-effect profiles of the available medications. For example, in a patient with hepatic disease, lithium is preferred because it does not require hepatic metabolism. For patients experiencing mixed episodes, valproate is preferred over lithium. Conventional antipsychotics should be avoided because they are associated with more extrapyramidal side effects and a greater risk of tardive dyskinesia compared with atypical antipsychotics. Antidepressants exacerbate mania and should be tapered and discontinued in patients who are manic or in a mixed state, even though depressive symptoms are present.

Although mood stabilizers are effective therapeutic agents, their efficacy may not be apparent for 1–2 weeks, occasionally longer. Because agitation and behavioral dyscontrol are often prominent in mania, additional medications are frequently used in the acute setting. The benzodiazepines lorazepam and clonazepam can be used to treat agitation and insomnia until the primary antimanic medication takes effect. Alprazolam is not recommended for patients with mania because, like all agents with antidepressant effects, it may precipitate mania (Arana et al. 1988).

When a patient fails to respond to a single agent, the next step is to combine medications. Adding a second agent is preferred to substituting one mood stabilizer for another, unless the patient had a toxic or an allergic reaction to the first drug. This strategy provides synergism and avoids the risk of exacerbating the patient's symptoms through withdrawal of the first agent, which, although seemingly ineffective, may have been providing some therapeutic benefit. After the patient is stabilized, it may be reasonable to consider tapering the dose of the first agent, although it is not unusual for patients with bipolar disorder to require long-term treatment with a combination of medications. Electroconvulsive therapy is an effective treatment for acute mania and is especially useful for patients who cannot safely wait until medication becomes effective.

■ TREATMENT OF BIPOLAR DEPRESSION

A common mistake is to treat bipolar depression in the same manner that one treats unipolar depression, overlooking the need for a mood stabilizer. In bipolar depression, the first pharmacological intervention should be to start or optimize treatment with a mood stabilizer rather than to start administering an antidepressant medication. In addition, thyroid function should be evaluated, particularly if the patient is taking lithium. Subclinical hypothyroidism, manifested as an increased thyroid-stimulating hormone level and normal triiodothyronine and thyroxine levels, may present as depression in affectively predisposed individuals. In such cases, the addition of thyroid hormones may be beneficial, even if there is no other evidence of hypothyroidism.

Lithium, lamotrigine, and olanzapine-fluoxetine combination therapy are first-line treatments for bipolar depression. The response rate to lithium in bipolar depression is 79% (Zornberg and Pope 1993). In a double-blind, placebo-controlled trial, lamotrigine was shown to be effective in patients with bipolar depression (Calabrese et al. 1999). Lamotrigine can be combined with other mood stabilizers, but it is important to remember that lamotrigine therapy is started at lower doses and dose titration is more gradual when this medication is added to valproate therapy. The combination of olanzapine and fluoxetine is particularly useful in patients who are not currently taking other psychiatric medications and who would benefit from a single pill rather than more traditional combined treatments. One study has reported efficacy of quetiapine monotherapy in bipolar depression (Calabrese et al. 2005). Data are less compelling regarding the use of valproate and carbamazepine for the acute treatment of bipolar depression. Hence if a patient is already taking valproate or carbamazepine, we recommend optimizing the dose and then considering adding either lithium or lamotrigine.

Some patients with bipolar disorder will need antidepressants. Although the switch rate into mania or induction of rapid cycling by antidepressants is controversial, these agents do appear to present a risk for some patients, often with devastating consequences. Therefore, when a patient with bipolar disorder is prescribed an antidepressant, it should only be in combination with a medication that has established antimanic properties. Controlled comparative data on the use of specific antidepressant drugs in the treatment of bipolar depression are sparse. Current treatment guidelines extrapolate from these few studies and rely heavily on anecdotal clinical experience. Overall, tricyclic antidepressants should be avoided when other viable treatment options exist. Electroconvulsive therapy should be considered in severe cases.

■ MAINTENANCE TREATMENT IN BIPOLAR DISORDER

Patients with bipolar disorder require lifelong prophylaxis with a mood stabilizer, both to prevent new episodes and to decrease the likelihood that the illness will become more severe. Ninety percent of bipolar patients relapse after stopping lithium therapy, most within 6 months (Suppes et al. 1991). In addition to the single episode that may occur, each episode may further kindle the illness, thereby inducing a more malignant course with decreased treatment responsiveness. The more episodes a patient has had, the less likely the disorder is to respond to treatment (Gelenberg et al. 1989).

An additional reason for continuing effective prophylactic treatment is the possibility of discontinuation-induced refractoriness (Post et al. 1992). Some patients who were previously treated with lithium successfully and who then have another episode after lithium has been discontinued fail to respond to retreatment with lithium. Moreover, these individuals tend to respond poorly to other treatments. Although discontinuation-induced refractoriness has been reported only with lithium, it is feasible that the phenomenon may occur with other agents. However, if tolerance develops, a period without the ineffective medication, along with institution of treatment with a different agent, is indicated. In most situations in which it is necessary to discontinue a mood stabilizer, tapering should be as slow as possible. Abruptly stopping lithium therapy is associated with a substantially higher rate of relapse than is tapering (Faedda et al. 1993). Again, although most currently available data relate to lithium, there is no reason to suspect that the principles differ for other mood stabilizers.

■ REFERENCES

American Psychiatric Association: Practice guideline for the treatment of patients with bipolar disorder (revision). Am J Psychiatry 159 (4 suppl): 1–50, 2002

Arana GW, Epstein S, Molloy M, et al: Carbamazepine-induced reduction of plasma alprazolam concentrations: a clinical case report. J Clin Psychiatry 49:448–449, 1988

Bertollini R, Kallen B, Mastroiacovo P, et al: Anticonvulsant drugs in monotherapy: effect on fetus. Eur J Epidemiol 3:164–171, 1987

Bowden CL, Janicak PG, Orsulak P, et al: Relation of serum valproate concentration to response in mania. Am J Psychiatry 153:765–770, 1996

Bowden CL, Calabrese JR, Sachs G, et al: A placebo-controlled 18-month trial of lamotrigine and lithium maintenance treatment in recently manic or hypomanic patients with bipolar I disorder. Lamictal 606 Study Group. Arch Gen Psychiatry 60:392–400, 2003

Bucht G, Smigan L, Wahlin A, et al: ECG changes during lithium therapy: a prospective study. Acta Med Scand 216:101–104, 1984

Calabrese JR, Bowden CL, Sachs GS, et al: A double-blind placebo-controlled study of lamotrigine monotherapy in outpatients with bipolar I depression. Lamictal 602 Study Group. J Clin Psychiatry 60:79–88, 1999

Calabrese JR, Suppes T, Bowden CL, et al: A double-blind, placebo-controlled, prophylaxis study of lamotrigine in rapid-cycling bipolar disorder. Lamictal 614 Study Group. J Clin Psychiatry 61:841–850, 2000

Calabrese JR, Bowden CL, Sachs GS, et al: A placebo-controlled 18-month trial of lamotrigine and lithium maintenance treatment in recently depressed patients with bipolar I disorder. Lamictal 605 Study Group. J Clin Psychiatry 64:1013–1024, 2003

Calabrese JR, Keck PE, Macfadden W, et al: A randomized, double-blind, placebo-controlled trial of quetiapine in the treatment of bipolar I or II depression. Am J Psychiatry 162:1351–1360, 2005

Chen G, Manji HK, Hawver DB, et al: Chronic sodium valproate selectively decreases protein kinase C alpha and epsilon in vitro. J Neurochem 63:2361–2364, 1994

Cohen LS, Friedman JM, Jefferson JW, et al: A reevaluation of risk of in utero exposure to lithium. JAMA 271:146–150, 1994

Coppen A, Abou-Saleh MT, Milln P, et al: Lithium continuation therapy following electroconvulsive therapy. Br J Psychiatry 139:284–287, 1981

Coyle JT, Duman RS: Finding the intracellular signaling pathways affected by mood disorder treatments. Neuron 38:157–160, 2003

Dean JC, Penry JK: Valproate, in The Medical Treatment of Epilepsy. Edited by Resor SR Jr, Kutt H. New York, Marcel Dekker, 1992, pp 265–278

Dunner DL, Fieve RR: Clinical factors in lithium carbonate prophylaxis failure. Arch Gen Psychiatry 30:229–233, 1974

Edmonds LD, Oakley GP: Ebstein's anomaly and maternal lithium exposure during pregnancy. Teratology 41:551–552, 1990

Emrich HM: Studies with oxcarbazepine (Trileptal) in acute mania. Int Clin Psychopharmacol 5:83–88, 1990

Faedda GL, Tondo L, Baldessarini RJ, et al: Outcome after rapid vs. gradual discontinuation of lithium treatment in bipolar disorders. Arch Gen Psychiatry 50:448–455, 1993

Frye MA, Ketter TA, Kimbrell TA, et al: A placebo-controlled study of lamotrigine and gabapentin monotherapy in refractory mood disorders. J Clin Psychopharmacol 20:607–614, 2000

Gelenberg AJ, Kane JM, Keller MB, et al: Comparison of standard and low serum levels of lithium for maintenance treatment of bipolar disorder. N Engl J Med 321:1489–1493, 1989

Gitlin MJ: Lithium-induced renal insufficiency. J Clin Psychopharmacol 13:276–279, 1993

Goldfrank LR, Lewin NA, Flomenbaum NE, et al: Antidepressants: tricyclics, tetracyclics, monoamine oxidase inhibitors, and others, in Goldfrank's Toxicologic Emergencies, 3rd Edition. Edited by Goldfrank LR, Flomenbaum NE, Lewin NA, et al. Norwalk, CT, Appleton-Century-Crofts, 1986, pp 351–363

Goodwin FK, Jamison R: Manic-Depressive Illness. New York, Oxford University Press, 1990

Hurd RW, Van Rinsvelt HA, Wilder BJ, et al: Selenium, zinc, and copper changes with valproic acid: possible relation to drug side effects. Neurology 34:1393–1395, 1984

Isojärvi JIT, Laatikainen TJ, Pakarinen AJ, et al: Polycystic ovaries and hyperandrogenism in women taking valproate for epilepsy. N Engl J Med 19:579–584, 1993

Isojärvi JI, Laatikainen TJ, Knip M, et al: Obesity and endocrine disorders in women taking valproate for epilepsy. Ann Neurol 39:579–584, 1996

Jacobsen FM: Low-dose valproate: a new treatment for cyclothymia, mild rapid cycling disorders, and premenstrual syndrome. J Clin Psychiatry 54:229–234, 1993

Jacobson SJ, Jones K, Johnson K, et al: Prospective multicentre study of pregnancy outcome after lithium exposure during first trimester. Lancet 339:530–533, 1992

Jaeken J, Casaer P, Corbeel L: Valproate, hyperammonaemia and hyperglycinaemia (letter). Lancet 2:260, 1980

Joffe H, Cohen LS, Suppes T, et al: Valproate is associated with new-onset oligoamenorrhea with hyperandrogenism in women with bipolar disorder. Biol Psychiatry (in press)

Jones KL, Lacro RV, Johnson KA, et al: Pattern of malformations in the children of women treated with carbamazepine during pregnancy. N Engl J Med 320:1661–1666, 1989

Kallen B, Tandberg A: Lithium and pregnancy: a cohort study in manic-depressive women. Acta Psychiatr Scand 68:134–139, 1983

Keck PE Jr, McElroy SL, Tugrul KC, et al: Valproate oral loading in the treatment of acute mania. J Clin Psychiatry 54:305–308, 1993

Ketter TA, Wang PW, Chandler RA, et al: Dermatology precautions and slower titration yield low incidence of lamotrigine treatment-emergent rash. J Clin Psychiatry 66:642–645, 2005

Kim JS, Chang MY, Yu IT, et al: Lithium selectivity increases neuronal differentiation of hippocampal neural progenitor cells both in vitro and in vivo. J Neurochem 89:324–336, 2004

Lammer EJ, Sever LE, Oakley GP Jr: Teratogen update: valproic acid. Teratology 35:465–473, 1987

Leach MJ, Baxter MG, Critchley MA: Neurochemical and behavioral aspects of lamotrigine. Epilepsia 32 (suppl 2):S4–S8, 1991

Lindstedt G, Nilsson L, Walinder J, et al: On the prevalence, diagnosis and management of lithium-induced hypothyroidism in psychiatric patients. Br J Psychiatry 130:452–458, 1977

Macdonald RL, Kelly KM: Antiepileptic drug mechanisms of action. Epilepsia 36:S2–S12, 1995

Manji HK, Chen G, Hsiao JK, et al: Regulation of signal transduction pathways by mood-stabilizing agents: implications for the delayed onset of therapeutic efficacy. J Clin Psychiatry 57 (suppl 13):34–46, 1996

Marangell LB, Martinez JM, Ketter TA, et al: Lamotrigine treatment of bipolar disorder: data from the first 500 patients in STEP-BD. Bipolar Disord 6:139–143, 2004

Markowitz GS, Radhakrishnan J, Kambham N, et al: Lithium nephrotoxicity: a progressive combined glomerular and tubulointerstitial nephropathy. J Am Soc Nephrol 11:1439–1448, 2000

Myers DH, Carter RA, Burns BH, et al: A prospective study of the effects of lithium on thyroid function and on the prevalence of antithyroid antibodies. Psychol Med 15:55–61, 1985

Pande AC, Crockatt JG, Janney CA, et al: Gabapentin in bipolar disorder: a placebo-controlled trial of adjunctive therapy. Gabapentin Bipolar Disorder Study Group. Bipolar Disord 2:249–255, 2000

Pellock JM, Willmore LJ: A rational guide to routine blood monitoring in patients receiving antiepileptic drugs. Neurology 41:961–964, 1991

Perlis RH, Sachs GS, Lafer B, et al: Effect of abrupt change from standard to low serum levels of lithium: a reanalysis of double-blind lithium maintenance data. Am J Psychiatry 159:1155–1159, 2002

Post RM, Leverich GS, Altshuler L, et al: Lithium-discontinuation-induced refractoriness: preliminary observations. Am J Psychiatry 149:1727–1729, 1992

Prien RF, Kupfer DJ, Mansky PA, et al: Drug therapy in the prevention of recurrences in unipolar and bipolar affective disorders: report of the NIMH Collaborative Study Group comparing lithium carbonate, imipramine, and a lithium carbonate-imipramine combination. Arch Gen Psychiatry 41:1096–1104, 1984

Robert E, Guibaud P: Maternal valproic acid and congenital neural tube defects (letter). Lancet 2:937, 1982

Rosa FW: Spina bifida in infants of women treated with carbamazepine during pregnancy. N Engl J Med 324:674–677, 1991

Sackeim HA, Haskett RF, Mulsant BH, et al: Continuation pharmacotherapy in the prevention of relapse following electroconvulsive therapy: a randomized controlled trial. JAMA 285:1299–1307, 2001

Suppes T, Baldessarini RJ, Faedda GL, et al: Risk of recurrence following discontinuation of lithium treatment in bipolar disorder. Arch Gen Psychiatry 48:1082–1088, 1991

Suppes T, Webb A, Paul B, et al: Clinical outcome in a randomized 1-year trial of clozapine versus treatment as usual for patients with treatment-resistant illness and a history of mania. Am J Psychiatry 156:1164–1169, 1999

Tohen M, Jacobs TG, Grundy SL, et al (Olanzapine HGGW Study Group): Efficacy of olanzapine in acute bipolar mania: a double-blind, placebo-controlled study. Arch Gen Psychiatry 57:841–849, 2000

Tohen M, Vieta E, Calabrese J, et al: Efficacy of olanzapine-fluoxetine combination in the treatment of bipolar I depression. Arch Gen Psychiatry 60:1079–1088, 2003

Wehr TA, Sack DA, Rosenthal NE, et al: Rapid cycling affective disorder: contributing factors and treatment responses in 51 patients. Am J Psychiatry 145:179–184, 1988

Weisler RH, Keck PE Jr, Swann AC, et al: Extended-release carbamazepine capsules as monotherapy for acute mania in bipolar disorder: a multicenter, randomized, double-blind, placebo-controlled trial. J Clin Psychiatry 66:323–330, 2005

Zalzstein E, Koren G, Einarson T, et al: A case-control study on the association between first trimester exposure to lithium and Ebstein's anomaly. Am J Cardiol 65:817–818, 1990

Zornberg GL, Pope HG Jr: Treatment of depression in bipolar disorder: new directions for research. J Clin Psychopharmacol 13:397–408, 1993

6

STIMULANTS

Stimulants are a class of psychoactive medications approved by the U.S. Food and Drug Administration (FDA) for use in the treatment of attention-deficit/hyperactivity disorder (ADHD) in children and adolescents and narcolepsy. A list of available stimulants is shown in Table 6–1.

■ MECHANISMS OF ACTION

Stimulants have putative effects on central dopaminergic and noradrenergic neurotransmission. Specifically, stimulants enhance dopamine synaptic transmission (Wilens and Biederman 1992). Methylphenidate stimulates the release of dopamine stores from vesicles in presynaptic neurons (Russell et al. 1998) and also may inhibit presynaptic dopamine reuptake and affect noradrenergic and serotonergic neurotransmission (Challman and Lipsky 2000). In animals, dextroamphetamine has been shown to block presynaptic dopamine and norepinephrine reuptake, inhibit monoamine oxidase, and facilitate catecholamine release (Homsi et al. 2000). Dextroamphetamine also has been shown to facilitate the release of dopamine from presynaptic neuron cytoplasmic stores (Masand and Tesar 1996). Pemoline blocks presynaptic dopamine reuptake in animals (Homsi et al. 2000). However, the exact mechanisms by which these agents complete their specific actions in treating ADHD have not been definitively established.

TABLE 6–1.   **Stimulant medications**

Drug	Trade name	Formulations
Methylphenidate	Ritalin	5-, 10-, 20-mg tablets
	Ritalin-SR	20-mg sustained-release tablets Must be taken whole
	Ritalin LA	10-, 20-, 30-, 40-mg extended-release capsules (can be opened and sprinkled over small amount of applesauce before immediate consumption)
	Methylin	5-, 10-, 20-mg tablets
	Methylin ER	10-, 20-mg tablets Must be taken whole
	Methylin Chewable	2.5-, 5-, 10-mg chewable tablets
	Methylin Oral solution	5 mg/5 mL, 10 mg/5 mL grape-flavored solutions
	Metadate ER	10-, 20-mg tablets Must be taken whole
	Metadate CD	10-, 20-, 30-mg capsules (can be opened and sprinkled over small amount of applesauce before immediate consumption)
	Concerta	18-, 27-, 36-, 54-mg extended-release tablets
Dexmethylphenidate	Focalin	2.5-, 5-, 10-mg tablets
	Focalin XR	5-, 10-, 20-mg extended-release capsules (can be opened and sprinkled over applesauce before immediate consumption)
Dextroamphetamine	Dexedrine	5-, 10-mg tablets
	DextroStat	5-, 10-mg tablets
	Dexedrine Spansule	5-, 10-, 15-mg sustained-release capsules

TABLE 6–1.	Stimulant medications *(continued)*	
Drug	**Trade name**	**Formulations**
Amphetamine/ dextroamphetamine	Adderall	5-, 7.5-, 10-, 12.5-, 15-, 20-, 30-mg tablets
	Adderall XR	5-, 10-, 15-, 20-, 25-, 30-mg extended-release capsules (can be opened and sprinkled over applesauce before immediate consumption)

Source. Adderall XR 2004; Focalin XR 2005; Fuller and Sajatovic 2000; Lee et al. 2003; Methylin Chewable Tablets 2004; Methylin Oral Solution 2004; Pentikis et al. 2002; Physicians' Desk Reference 2005a, 2005b; Tulloch et al. 2002.

■ PHARMACOKINETICS

Stimulants are rapidly absorbed from the gastrointestinal tract after oral administration, rapidly metabolized, and excreted mainly in the urine. They are not highly protein bound, but they are lipophilic and, therefore, cross the blood-brain barrier and the placenta.

■ CONTRAINDICATIONS

Contraindications to stimulant use include a history of hypersensitivity to the particular agent, significant cardiovascular disease, moderate to severe uncontrolled hypertension, hyperthyroidism, marked anxiety or agitation, glaucoma, a history of drug abuse, and concomitant use of monoamine oxidase inhibitors (MAOIs). A personal history of motor tics or a family history of Tourette's syndrome are also reported as contraindications to the use of stimulants because some children with ADHD may experience new tics or worsening of preexisting tics. However, some clinicians argue that stimulants may be used if the potential benefits outweigh the risks, provided that other treatment options are considered and the patient is closely monitored for the presence or worsening of tics. Patients with active psychosis should not be administered stimulants because these agents may exacerbate psychotic symptoms.

■ RISKS, SIDE EFFECTS, AND THEIR MANAGEMENT

A partial list of stimulant side effects is outlined in Table 6–2. Common side effects (such as insomnia, nervousness, nausea, decreased appetite, stomachaches, and headaches) tend to be transient and diminish with time or medication discontinuation. Using the lowest effective dose, taking the medications with meals, and avoiding doses late in the day help minimize these side effects as well.

"Rebound" symptoms, including irritability and hyperactivity, have been described and may occur as plasma concentrations decrease after the last daily dose. Management of rebound symptoms may include using a small dose of medication in the late afternoon or switching to a long-acting preparation.

Withdrawal symptoms, more commonly seen in individuals who chronically abuse high doses of stimulants, include increased sleep with vivid dreams, increased appetite, fatigue, and drug craving.

Sudden deaths have occurred with amphetamine use in children with cardiac abnormalities, and clinicians are cautioned against administering amphetamine stimulants to patients with structural cardiac abnormalities.

■ OVERDOSE

Overdose of stimulants may lead to signs and symptoms of sympathetic overstimulation, including tremors, hypertension, fever, tachycardia, hyperreflexia, confusion, agitation, and frank psychosis or delirium. Management typically involves supportive measures to treat fever, severe hypertension, seizures, agitation, and other signs and symptoms.

■ ABUSE

In general, clinicians should closely monitor the use of stimulants and be aware of the risks of potential abuse by patients and those around them, including family members, friends, and school personnel responsible for dispensing medications. One should exercise

TABLE 6–2.   **Potential side effects of stimulants**

General

Delayed growth   Sweating

HEENT

Headache   Blurred vision

Cardiovascular

Tachycardia   Hypotension
Bradycardia   Chest pain
Hypertension   Palpitations

Gastrointestinal

Nausea   Decreased appetite
Vomiting   Weight loss
Dry mouth   Abdominal pain

Dermatological

Rash   Pruritis

Neurological

Nervousness   Tics
Insomnia   Tremor
Movement disorders   Euphoria
Restlessness   Dysphoria
Anxiety   Psychosis
Agitation   Seizures
Drowsiness   Gilles de la Tourette's syndrome
Dizziness   Neuroleptic malignant syndrome

Note. HEENT=head, ears, eyes, nose, and throat.
Source. Fuller and Sajatovic 2000; Lee et al. 2003, Pentikis et al. 2002; Physicians' Desk Reference 2005a.

great caution when considering treatment with stimulants in any patient with a history of substance abuse or dependence. These agents are contraindicated in patients with a history of stimulant drug abuse.

■ DOSING

Stimulants are available in several formulations, with durations of action in ADHD ranging from 3 to 12 hours. The approximate time

TABLE 6–3. Pharmacokinetic properties and approximate durations of action of stimulants

Drug	Trade name	Time to peak plasma concentration (hours)	Half-life (mean hours)	Duration of action in ADHD (hours)[a]
Methylphenidate	Ritalin, Methylin	1–2	2–4	4
	Ritalin-SR, Methylin ER, Metadate ER	4.7	3–4	6–8
	Ritalin LA	1–3 (initial peak) 5–11 (second peak)	2.5 (children) 3.5 (adults)	8–9
	Metadate CD	1.5 (initial peak) 4.5 (second peak)	6.8	8–9
	Concerta	1–2 (initial peak) 6–8 (second peak)	3.5	10–12
Dexmethylphenidate	Focalin	1–1.5	2.2	4–6
	Focalin XR	1.5 (initial peak) 6.5 (second peak)	2–3 (children) 2–4.5 (adults)	>6
Dextroamphetamine	Dexedrine, Dextrostat	2–3	10.5–12	4
	Dexedrine Spansule	8	12	6–8

TABLE 6–3. Pharmacokinetic properties and approximate durations of action of stimulants *(continued)*

Drug	Trade name	Time to peak plasma concentration (hours)	Half-life (mean hours)	Duration of action in ADHD (hours)[a]
Amphetamine/ dextroamphetamine	Adderall	3	D-amphetamine: 9.7–11 L-amphetamine: 11–13.8	Dose-dependent: 3.5 (5-mg dose) 6.4 (20-mg dose)
	Adderall XR	7	D-amphetamine: 10 (adults) 9 (children) L-amphetamine: 13 (adults) 11 (children)	10–12

Note. ADHD=attention-deficit/hyperactivity disorder.

[a]Times are approximate and may vary from patient to patient.

Source. Adderall XR 2004; Arnold et al. 2004; Biederman and Faraone 2005; Connor and Steingard 2004; Green 2001; McGough et al. 2005a, 2005b; Pelham et al. 1999; Physicians' Desk Reference 2005a, 2005b; Santosh and Taylor 2000; Swanson and Volkow 2002; Swanson et al. 2004; Wigal et al. 2004.

to onset of action and duration of action for the various stimulants are given in Table 6–3. Dosing strategies for the treatment of ADHD and narcolepsy are outlined in Table 6–4.

■ MONITORING GUIDELINES

At baseline and throughout treatment, the patient's target symptoms, blood pressure, pulse, height, weight, and appetite should be evaluated, and growth charts should be maintained (Greenhill et al. 2002b; Santosh and Taylor 2000). Because of the risk of hematological abnormalities, complete blood cell counts with differential analyses should be monitored periodically as well. The clinician also should evaluate for the onset or exacerbation of tics or dyskinesias.

■ STIMULANT MEDICATIONS

Methylphenidate

Methylphenidate hydrochloride, a piperidine derivative structurally similar to amphetamine, is a commonly prescribed stimulant for the treatment of ADHD in children age 6 years and older. It is a racemic mixture of *d,l* methyl α-phenyl-2-piperidineacetate hydrochloride. The drug is available in immediate-release, extended-release, and controlled-release formulations. It is hepatically metabolized to an inactive metabolite and excreted by the kidneys.

In school-age children and adolescents with ADHD, treatment with immediate-release methylphenidate typically consists of administration once a day in the morning or in divided morning and noon doses. Doses can then be titrated upward on a weekly basis until improvement of target symptoms is achieved. Some patients take a third dose (typically 50% of other doses) in the late afternoon to manage symptoms in the early evening hours or to minimize rebound symptoms. Extended-release and controlled-release formulations have longer durations of action and are often preferred because less frequent dosing is needed.

TABLE 6-4. Dosing strategies for stimulants

Drug	Trade name	General dosing strategies
Methylphenidate	Ritalin, Methylin	*ADHD and narcolepsy:* Children ≥6 years old: Start at 5 mg qam or bid; increase by 5–10 mg/day at weekly intervals as needed to attain response. Give three times daily if effect is needed in evening hours. Maximum total daily dose: 60 mg Adults: Start at 5–10 mg bid; titrate as above.
	Ritalin-SR, Methylin ER, Metadate ER	*ADHD:* May be given once every morning in place of total daily dose of immediate-release methylphenidate to achieve an estimated 8-hour duration of action. Must be taken whole.
	Ritalin LA	*ADHD:* Children ≥6 years old: Start at 20 mg once daily (or lower at clinician's discretion); increase by 10 mg weekly. *Switching from immediate-release methylphenidate or methylphenidate-SR:* Start Ritalin LA at total daily dose of immediate-release methylphenidate or methylphenidate-SR (administer Ritalin LA dose once daily). Maximum total daily dose: 60 mg
	Metadate CD	*ADHD:* Persons ≥6 years old: start at 20 mg qam; increase by 10–20 mg/day at weekly intervals as needed to attain response. Maximum total daily dose: 60 mg

TABLE 6–4.   Dosing strategies for stimulants *(continued)*

Drug	Trade name	General dosing strategies
Methylphenidate *(continued)*	Concerta	*ADHD:* Persons ≥6 years old: Start at 18 mg qam; increase by 18 mg/day at weekly intervals.
		Maximum total daily dose: 54 mg
		Switching from other methylphenidate preparations:
		Begin Concerta 18 mg qam if administering methylphenidate 5 mg bid or tid or methylphenidate-SR 20 mg/day.
		Begin Concerta 36 mg qam if administering methylphenidate 10 mg bid or tid or methylphenidate-SR 40 mg/day.
		Begin Concerta 54 mg qam if administering methylphenidate 15 mg bid or tid or methylphenidate-SR 60 mg/day.
		Maximum total daily dose: 54 mg (some adolescents may be titrated to a maximum of 72 mg/day, not to exceed 2 mg/kg body weight/day).
		Must be taken whole.
Dexmethylphenidate	Focalin	*ADHD:* Persons ≥6 years old: start at 2.5 mg bid; increase by 2.5–5 mg/day at weekly intervals.
		Switching from immediate-release methylphenidate: Start Focalin at 50% of the methylphenidate dose (administer Focalin in divided bid doses); titrate as above.
		Maximum total daily dose: 10 mg bid

TABLE 6–4. Dosing strategies for stimulants (continued)

Drug	Trade name	General dosing strategies
Dexmethylphenidate (continued)	Focalin XR	*ADHD:* Children ≥5 years old: Start at 5 mg/day; increase by 5 mg/day at weekly intervals. Adults: Start at 10 mg/day; increase by 10 mg/day at weekly intervals. *Switching from methylphenidate:* Start Focalin XR at 50% of the total daily dose of methylphenidate (administer Focalin XR in a once-daily dose); titrate Focalin XR as above. *Switching from immediate-release dexmethylphenidate (Focalin):* Start Focalin XR at the same total daily dose as the Focalin dose. Maximum total daily dose: 20 mg (children and adults)
Dextroamphetamine	Dexedrine, DextroStat	*ADHD:* Children 3–5 years old: Start at 2.5 mg qam; increase by 2.5 mg/day at weekly intervals. Children ≥6 years old: Start at 5 mg qam or bid; increase by 5 mg/day at weekly intervals. Maximum total daily dose: 40 mg *Narcolepsy:* Children 6–12 years old: Start at 5 mg/day; increase by 5 mg/day at weekly intervals. Persons >12 years old: Start at 10 mg/day; increase by 10 mg/day at weekly intervals. Maximum total daily dose: 60 mg

TABLE 6–4. Dosing strategies for stimulants *(continued)*

Drug	Trade name	General dosing strategies
Dextroamphetamine *(continued)*	Dexedrine Spansule	Dosing similar to Dexedrine dosing, except use once-daily dosing when appropriate.
Amphetamine/ dextroamphetamine	Adderall	*ADHD:* Children 3–5 years old: Start at 2.5 mg qam; increase by 2.5 mg/day at weekly intervals. Children≥6 years old: Start at 5 mg qam or bid; increase by 5 mg/day at weekly intervals. Maximum total daily dose: 40 mg *Narcolepsy:* Children 6–12 years old: Start at 5 mg/day; increase by 5 mg/day at weekly intervals. Persons>12 years old: Start at 10 mg/day; increase by 10 mg/day at weekly intervals.
	Adderall XR	*ADHD:* Children≥6 years old: Start at 10 mg qam; increase by 5–10 mg/day at weekly intervals. Adults: Recommended dose is 20 mg/day.

TABLE 6–4. Dosing strategies for stimulants *(continued)*

Drug	Trade name	General dosing strategies
Amphetamine/ dextroamphetamine *(continued)*		Maximum total daily dose: 30 mg *Switching from immediate-release Adderall:* Switch to the same total daily dose (administer Adderall XR once daily). No studies in children <6 years old.

Note. ADHD=attention/deficit/hyperactivity disorder; qam=every morning; bid=twice daily; SR=sustained release; tid=three times a day; ALT=alanine aminotransferase.

Source. Adderall XR 2004; Focalin XR 2005; Fuller and Sajatovic 2000; Physicians' Desk Reference 2005a; Spencer et al. 2003.

Several different long-acting methylphenidate preparations are shown in Table 6–5. The reader should note the differences in pharmacokinetics and drug delivery mechanisms between these agents (Tables 6–3 and 6–5). Head-to-head comparisons of pharmacokinetic profiles have been done between Concerta and Metadate CD (Gonzalez et al. 2002) and between Concerta and Ritalin LA (Markowitz et al. 2003). Pharmacokinetic differences between agents may translate into clinically meaningful differences, as some data suggest that long-acting methylphenidate preparations may differ in their relative patterns of efficacy (but not overall efficacy) at different time points during the day (Lopez et al. 2003; Swanson et al. 2004). Specifically, some formulations deliver 50% of their total methylphenidate dose immediately, whereas others deliver a lower percentage of methylphenidate early but a greater percentage of drug later (see the following paragraphs and Table 6–5). Thus, some patients may benefit from a higher methylphenidate dose in the morning, but others may benefit from receiving a greater dose in the afternoon. Of course, individual responses to these agents may vary.

Extended-release and sustained-release tablets are more slowly absorbed than immediate-release methylphenidate and provide up to an 8-hour duration of action (Table 6–3), although some clinicians believe that their initial onset of action is delayed compared with immediate-release preparations (Pelham et al. 1987; Swanson and Volkow 2002). Concerta, a preparation that contains 22% of the medication in an immediate-release tablet overcoat and uses an osmotic process to deliver the remainder of the methylphenidate at a controlled rate, may be effective for up to a 12-hour period and may be used as a substitute for three-times-daily immediate-release methylphenidate (Modi et al. 2000a, 2000b; Pelham et al. 2001; Spencer et al. 2003; Swanson et al. 2003; Wolraich et al. 2001). Because this formulation uses an osmotic release delivery system, patients should be advised to remain adequately hydrated to ensure appropriate drug delivery. Metadate CD, a preparation that provides 30% of the methylphenidate dose by immediate-release beads and 70% by extended-release beads, is reported to have an 8-hour duration of action (Greenhill et al. 2002a; Physicians' Desk Reference 2005a).

TABLE 6–5.   Drug delivery systems of long-acting stimulant formulations

Drug	Trade name	Drug delivery system
Methylphenidate	Ritalin-SR	Slowly absorbed tablet
	Ritalin LA	Capsule with 50% methylphenidate dose as immediate-release beads and 50% as delayed-release beads
	Metadate ER	Slowly absorbed tablet with methylphenidate incorporated in a wax matrix tablet, allowing gradual diffusion
	Metadate CD	Capsule that provides 30% of methylphenidate dose by immediate-release beads and 70% of the dose by extended-release beads
	Concerta	Tablet that contains approximately 22% of the methylphenidate dose in an immediate-release capsule overcoat and 78% within the tablet that is released by an osmotic process over an extended period
Dexmethylphenidate	Focalin XR	Capsule with 50% dexmethylphenidate dose as immediate-release beads and 50% as delayed-release beads
Dextroamphetamine	Dexedrine Spansule	Capsule that allows some medication release immediately and the remainder released over time
Amphetamine/ dextroamphetamine	Adderall XR	Capsule with a 50:50 mixture of immediate-release beads and delayed-release beads, designed to provide treatment for 12 hours

Source.   Adderall XR 2004; Connor and Steingard 2004; Focalin XR 2005; Physicians' Desk Reference 2005a; Ritalin LA 2004.

Ritalin LA, which contains half the methylphenidate dose in immediate-release beads and half the dose in enteric-coated, delayed-release beads, is also intended to provide efficacy throughout at least the school day (Biederman et al. 2003; Lopez et al. 2003).

Dexmethylphenidate is the *d*-threo-enantiomer of methylphenidate (Wigal et al. 2004). It is currently available in two formulations in the United States: Focalin and Focalin XR. Focalin is an immediate-release preparation with a plasma half-life of approximately 2.2 hours. Its duration of action is similar to, or possibly slightly longer (6 hours) than, that of immediate-release methylphenidate (Arnold et al. 2004; Wigal et al. 2004); thus, dosing is recommended twice daily. Focalin is approved by the FDA for the treatment of ADHD in children age 6 years and older. Focalin XR is an extended-release formulation in which capsules contain half of the dexmethylphenidate dose in immediate-release beads and half of the dose in delayed-release beads. Focalin XR produces two distinct plasma concentration peaks: at approximately 1.5 hours and 6.5 hours after a single daily dose (Focalin XR 2005). Focalin XR is approved for the treatment of ADHD in adults, adolescents, and children age 6 years and older.

Drug Interactions

Methylphenidate may decrease therapeutic effects of concomitantly administered antihypertensive medications and may potentiate effects of warfarin, phenytoin, phenylbutazone, and tricyclic antidepressants. When methylphenidate and MAOIs are coadministered, hypertensive crisis may result.

Dextroamphetamine

Dextroamphetamine, the *d*-isomer of amphetamine, is available in immediate-release and extended-release formulations. It is functionally more potent than methylphenidate and may be associated with a greater risk of growth retardation and abuse.

Amphetamine/dextroamphetamine (Adderall) is also more potent than methylphenidate, and it has a longer half-life. It is a mixture of four amphetamine salts: dextroamphetamine saccharate, dextro-amphetamine sulfate, amphetamine aspartate, and amphetamine sulfate. Adderall XR, an extended-release formulation that has immediate- and extended-release beads to deliver the medication, reaches peak plasma concentrations in 7 hours and has a half-life of approximately 9–11 hours in children and 10–13 hours in adults (Adderall XR 2004). It is approved by the FDA for the treatment of ADHD in children ages 6–12 years, adolescents, and adults. This long-acting formulation is bioequivalent to a similar total dose of amphetamine/dextroamphetamine administered twice daily (Tulloch et al. 2002) and may provide effects in ADHD over a 12-hour period (Biederman et al. 2002; McCracken et al. 2003).

Drug Interactions

The risk of tachycardia, hypertension, and cardiotoxicity is increased with coadministration of dronabinol (an antiemetic) and dextroamphetamine. In addition, administration of dextroamphetamine with MAOIs may increase the risk of hypertensive crisis. Alkalinizing agents can speed absorption (e.g., antacids) or delay urinary excretion (e.g., acetazolamide, thiazide diuretics) of dextroamphetamine, thus potentiating its effects. Gastric or urinary acidifying agents (e.g., ascorbic acid, ammonium chloride) can decrease the effects of dextroamphetamine. Propoxyphene overdose can potentiate amphetamine central nervous system stimulation, potentially resulting in fatal convulsions.

Pemoline

Pemoline is an oxazolidinone derivative that is not structurally similar to amphetamine or methylphenidate. It has fewer stimulating properties than other stimulants and may have less abuse potential. Unlike most other stimulants, pemoline is a Schedule IV agent and does not require a triplicate prescription. However, there are numerous reports of hepatotoxicity in patients taking pemoline (see review by Safer et al. 2001), and it is no longer available in the United States.

Modafinil

Modafinil is a stimulant medication used to improve wakefulness in patients with narcolepsy, obstructive sleep apnea/hypopnea syndrome (as adjunct to standard treatments for the underlying disorder), and shift work sleep disorder. Controlled and open trials provided data on the efficacy and safety of modafinil in patients with narcolepsy (Besset et al. 1996; Billiard et al. 1994; Broughton et al. 1997; Mitler et al. 2000; U.S. Modafinil in Narcolepsy Multicenter Study Group 1998, 2000). Modafinil has a long duration of action and low potential for dependence and may be a reasonable first choice in the treatment of mild to moderate narcolepsy (Silber 2001). There is also considerable interest in the potential use of modafinil in the treatment of ADHD, and studies are in progress.

Modafinil is a Schedule IV medication and does not require a triplicate prescription. Its mechanism of action is unclear but is thought to differ from those of conventional stimulants. Modafinil is metabolized by the liver and excreted by the kidneys. Its half-life is approximately 15 hours. It is available in 100- and 200-mg tablets. The typical daily dose is 200–400 mg every morning; this dose should be reduced in elderly or hepatically impaired patients.

Contraindications

Modafinil is contraindicated in patients with a known hypersensitivity to it, and the drug should be used cautiously in patients with a history of psychosis or cardiovascular disease.

Side Effects

Side effects are similar to those of other stimulants. Additionally, some patients may experience confusion, ataxia, hyperglycemia, gingival ulcers, urinary retention, paresthesias, neck and joint discomfort, amblyopia, pharyngitis, or dyspnea.

Drug Interactions

Modafinil is a substrate for the cytochrome P450 (CYP) enzyme 3A4. It is also induces CYP 1A2, 2B6, and 3A4 and can decrease the serum levels and effectiveness of substrates for these enzymes, including oral contraceptives. It is an inhibitor of CYP 2C9 and 2C19 and can increase serum levels of their substrates.

■ TREATMENT OF SPECIFIC DISORDERS

Attention-Deficit/Hyperactivity Disorder

More than 150 studies involving thousands of subjects (predominantly school-age children) have shown the efficacy of stimulants in the short-term treatment of ADHD in children. Stimulants have been reported to be effective in improving various symptom domains in ADHD, including inattention, impulsivity, hyperactivity, and oppositional or disruptive behavior. They have also been reported to improve parent-child and peer interactions, problem solving during games with peers, short-term memory, and reaction time. Clinically meaningful response rates among school-age children and adolescents with ADHD are reported at 70% or higher (Spencer et al. 1996). However, a positive response to stimulants in and of itself is not diagnostic of ADHD because stimulants may improve behavior in nonaffected children as well (Rapoport et al. 1980).

When selecting an initial stimulant agent, methylphenidate, dexmethylphenidate, dextroamphetamine, or amphetamine mixed salts formulations can be considered first line options. A patient with ADHD is typically first given a low dose of a particular agent, and the dose is titrated upward on a weekly basis to the lowest effective dose. Doses are individualized according to clinical response because correlations between plasma levels and response have not been established. Clinician-, teacher-, and parent-rated scales can be used to monitor target symptoms and their response to treatment. All currently available stimulants are thought to be equally effective in treating ADHD, although individuals' symptoms may respond preferentially to a particular agent. Therefore, if a patient's symptoms do not respond to an initial stimulant, trials of different stimulants are indicated before a switch is made to a different medication class. Tolerance to therapeutic effects in ADHD is unusual. Practice guidelines recommend weekly contact with patients during the initial titration phase of treatment and during periods of dosage adjustments (Greenhill et al. 2002b).

Narcolepsy

Some stimulants are approved for treatment of narcolepsy. Stimulants mainly improve excessive daytime sleepiness, and the effects may be dose related (Mitler et al. 1990). However, cataplexy usually does not respond to stimulants (Hyman et al. 1995). Stimulants are often administered in divided daily doses, and doses are often titrated weekly on the basis of clinical response.

■ OTHER POTENTIAL USES OF STIMULANTS

There also has been great interest in the use of stimulants to treat depressive symptoms. Small case series suggest the potential usefulness of adding stimulants to antidepressant therapy in treatment-resistant depression (Masand et al. 1998; Stoll et al. 1996). Stimulants also have been used in the treatment of depressive symptoms in medically ill elderly patients (see reviews by Challman and Lipsky 2000 and Masand and Tesar 1996). Short-term use of stimulants may rapidly improve symptoms of apathy and social withdrawal in these patients.

Methylphenidate has been shown to have therapeutic effects on depressive symptoms and cognitive functioning in cancer patients (Fernandez et al. 1987; Macleod 1998; Meyers et al. 1998; Olin and Masand 1996). In addition, some case reports and uncontrolled trials suggested a role for stimulants in treating cognitive impairment and depressive symptoms in patients with acquired immunodeficiency syndrome (Angrist et al. 1992; Fernandez et al. 1988a, 1988b; Holmes et al. 1989).

■ NONSTIMULANT MEDICATION FOR ATTENTION-DEFICIT/HYPERACTIVITY DISORDER

Atomoxetine

Atomoxetine is a nonstimulant medication approved by the U.S. FDA for the treatment of ADHD in children older than 6 years, adolescents, and adults. Numerous studies have confirmed its efficacy in the treatment of ADHD (Heiligenstein et al. 2000; Kelsey et al. 2004; Kratochvil et al. 2001, 2002; Michelson et al. 2001, 2002, 2003, 2004; Spencer et al. 1998, 2001, 2002). Atomoxetine provides clinicians with a nonstimulant pharmacological intervention for patients with ADHD who have not had good outcomes with stimulants because of poor efficacy or tolerability, as well as for patients in whom the abuse potential of stimulants is of particular concern.

Mechanism of Action

Atomoxetine is a selective inhibitor of norepinephrine presynaptic reuptake transporters that has been shown to increase extracellular norepinephrine and dopamine concentrations in the prefrontal cortex in rats (Bymaster et al. 2002), which may account for its clinical efficacy in the treatment of ADHD symptomatology. However, atomoxetine does not appear to affect dopamine levels in the striatum or nucleus accumbens and consequently is not thought to carry the abuse potential associated with stimulant medications.

Pharmacokinetics

Atomoxetine is rapidly absorbed after oral administration, is highly protein bound, and reaches peak plasma concentrations in 1–2 hours (Farid et al. 1985). It is primarily metabolized by the CYP 2D6 isoenzyme, and its half-life differs between "extensive 2D6 metabolizers" and "poor 2D6 metabolizers" (5.2 hours and 21.6 hours, respectively) (Farid et al. 1985).

Contraindications

Atomoxetine is contraindicated in patients with narrow-angle glaucoma or in combination with an MAOI.

Side Effects

Available safety data come from short-term trials of atomoxetine in the treatment of ADHD. Common side effects in studies of atomoxetine in children and adolescents include headache, upper abdominal pain, decreased appetite, nausea, vomiting, irritability, and dizziness (Wernicke and Kratochvil 2002). Other side effects observed in clinical trials of adults include constipation, somnolence, dry mouth, insomnia, urinary hesitancy and/or retention, and impaired sexual function. Postmarketing reports suggest that atomoxetine may cause severe liver injury in rare cases.

Atomoxetine also may increase heart rate and blood pressure and should be used with caution in patients with hypertension, tachycardia, cardiovascular disease, or cerebrovascular disease. Orthostatic hypotension also has been reported with atomoxetine therapy.

Children and adolescents taking atomoxetine should be monitored for the appearance or worsening of aggressive or hostile behavior because these symptoms were noted more frequently in children and adolescents taking atomoxetine than in those taking placebo in clinical trials (Strattera 2005).

Additionally, current product labeling contains a boxed warning regarding an increased risk of suicidal ideation in children and adolescents. Pooled analyses of 12 short-term atomoxetine trials showed an average risk of suicidal ideation of 0.4% in patients taking atomoxetine, compared with none in patients receiving placebo (Strattera 2005). Patients should be advised of the risks associated with atomoxetine prior to treatment.

Drug Interactions

Atomoxetine has not been shown to exert clinically significant inhibition of CYP 1A2, CYP 2C9, CYP 2D6, and CYP 3A isoenzymes (Sauer et al. 2004). However, paroxetine, a potent CYP 2D6 inhibitor, has been shown to increase plasma concentrations of atomoxetine and significantly increase the half-life of atomoxetine approximately 2.5-fold in "extensive 2D6 metabolizers" (Belle et al. 2002). Caution should be used when administering atomoxetine to patients taking albuterol or pressor agents because atomoxetine may potentiate the cardiovascular effects of albuterol or pressor agents.

Dosing

Atomoxetine is available in 10-, 18-, 25-, 40-, and 60-mg capsules. Dosing recommendations vary according to patient age and weight. In children and adolescents who weigh less than 70 kg, atomoxetine should be started at a total daily dose of 0.5 mg/kg body weight and increased after a minimum of 3 days to a target daily dose of 1.2 mg/kg (either as a single morning dose or divided evenly into morning and late afternoon doses), not to exceed a total daily dose of the lesser of 1.4 mg/kg body weight or 100 mg. In patients who weigh more than 70 kg, atomoxetine can be started at a total daily dose of 40 mg and increased after a minimum of 3 days to a total daily dose of 80 mg. Product labeling provides additional dosing recommendations in special populations, including those with hepatic impairment and those taking potent CYP 2D6 inhibitors.

■ REFERENCES

Adderall XR (package insert). Wayne, PA, Shire US Inc, 2004

Angrist B, d'Hollosy M, Sanfilipo M, et al: Central nervous system stimulants as symptomatic treatments for AIDS-related neuropsychiatric impairment. J Clin Psychopharmacol 12:268–272, 1992

Arnold LE, Lindsay RL, Connors CK, et al: A double-blind, placebo-controlled withdrawal trial of dexmethylphenidate hydrochloride in children with attention-deficit hyperactivity disorder. J Am Acad Child Adolesc Psychiatry 14:542–554, 2004

Belle DJ, Ernest CS, Sauer JM, et al: Effect of potent CYP2D6 inhibition by paroxetine on atomoxetine pharmacokinetics. J Clin Pharmacol 42:1219–1227, 2002

Besset A, Chetrit M, Carlander B, et al: Use of modafinil in the treatment of narcolepsy: a long-term follow-up study. Neurophysiol Clin 26:60–66, 1996

Biederman J, Faraone SV: Attention-deficit hyperactivity disorder. Lancet 366:237–248, 2005

Biederman J, Lopez FA, Boellner SW, et al: A randomized, double-blind, placebo-controlled, parallel-group study of SLI381 (Adderall XR) in children with attention-deficit/hyperactivity disorder. Pediatrics 110:258–266, 2002

Biederman J, Quinn D, Weiss M, et al: Efficacy and safety of Ritalin LA, a new, once daily, extended-release dosage form of methylphenidate, in children with attention deficit hyperactivity disorder. Paediatr Drugs 5:833–841, 2003

Billiard M, Besset A, Montplaisir J, et al: Modafinil: a double-blind multicenter study. Sleep 17:S107–S112, 1994

Broughton RJ, Fleming JA, George CF, et al: Randomized, double-blind, placebo-controlled crossover trial of modafinil in the treatment of excessive daytime sleepiness in narcolepsy. Neurology 49:444–451, 1997

Bymaster FP, Katner JS, Nelson DL, et al: Atomoxetine increases extracellular levels of norepinephrine and dopamine in prefrontal cortex of rat: a potential mechanism for efficacy in attention-deficit/hyperactivity disorder. Neuropsychopharmacology 27:699–711, 2002

Challman TD, Lipsky JJ: Methylphenidate: its pharmacology and uses. Mayo Clin Proc 75:711–721, 2000

Connor DF, Steingard RJ: New formulations of stimulants for attention deficit hyperactivity disorder: therapeutic potential. CNS Drugs 14:1011–1030, 2004

Farid NA, Bergstrom RF, Ziege EA, et al: Single-dose and steady-state pharmacokinetics of tomoxetine in normal subjects. J Clin Pharmacol 25:296–301, 1985

Fernandez F, Adams F, Holmes VF, et al: Methylphenidate for depressive disorders in cancer patients: an alternative to standard antidepressants. Psychosomatics 28:455–461, 1987

Fernandez F, Adams F, Levy JK, et al: Cognitive impairment due to AIDS-related complex and its response to psychostimulants. Psychosomatics 29:38–46, 1988a

Fernandez F, Levy JK, Galizzi H: Response of HIV-related depression to psychostimulants: case reports. Hosp Community Psychiatry 39:628–631, 1988b

Focalin XR (package insert). East Hanover, NJ, Novartis Pharmaceutical Corp, 2005

Fuller MA, Sajatovic M: Psychotropic Drug Information Handbook. Hudson, OH, Lexi-Comp, 2000

Gonzalez MA, Pentkis HS, Anderi N, et al: Methylphenidate bioavailability from two extended-release formulations. Int J Clin Pharmacol Ther 40:175–184, 2002

Green WH: Child and Adolescent Clinical Psychopharmacology, 3rd Edition. Philadelphia, PA, Lippincott Williams & Wilkins, 2001

Greenhill LL, Findling RL, Swanson JM, et al: A double-blind, placebo-controlled study of modified-release methylphenidate in children with attention-deficit/hyperactivity disorder. Pediatrics 109:E39, 2002a

Greenhill LL, Pliszka S, Dulcan MK, et al: Practice parameters for the use of stimulant medications in the treatment of children, adolescents, and adults. J Am Acad Child Adolesc Psychiatry 41 (2 suppl):26S–49S, 2002b

Heiligenstein J, Spencer T, Faries DE, et al: Efficacy of atomoxetine versus placebo in pediatric outpatients with ADHD. Presented at the 47th annual meeting of the American Academy of Child and Adolescent Psychiatry, New York, October 2000

Holmes VF, Fernandez F, Levy JK: Psychostimulant response in AIDS-related complex patients. J Clin Psychiatry 50:5–8, 1989

Homsi J, Walsh D, Nelson KA: Psychostimulants in supportive care. Support Care Cancer 8:385–397, 2000

Hyman SE, Arana GW, Rosenbaum JF: Handbook of Psychiatric Drug Therapy, 3rd Edition. Boston, MA, Little, Brown, 1995

Kelsey DK, Sumner CR, Casat CD, et al: Once-daily atomoxetine for children with attention-deficit/hyperactivity disorder, including an assessment of evening and morning behavior: a double-blind, placebo-controlled trial. Pediatrics 114:1–8, 2004

Kratochvil CJ, Bohac D, Harrington M, et al: An open-label trial of atomoxetine in pediatric attention deficit hyperactivity disorder. J Child Adolesc Psychopharmacol 11:167–170, 2001

Kratochvil CJ, Heiligenstein JH, Dittmann R, et al: Atomoxetine and methylphenidate treatment in children with ADHD: a prospective, randomized, open-label trial. J Am Acad Child Adolesc Psychiatry 41:776–784, 2002

Lee L, Kepple J, Wang Y, et al: Bioavailability of modified-release methylphenidate: influence of high-fat breakfast when administered intact and when capsule content sprinkled on applesauce. Biopharm Drug Dispos 24:233–243, 2003

Lopez F, Silva R, Pestreich L, et al: Comparative efficacy of two once daily methylphenidate formulations (Ritalin LA and Concerta) and placebo in children with attention-deficit hyperactivity disorder across the school day. Paediatr Drugs 5:545–555, 2003

Macleod AD: Methylphenidate in terminal depression. J Pain Symptom Manage 16:193–198, 1998

Markowitz JS, Straughn AB, Patrick KS, et al: Pharmacokinetics of methylphenidate after oral administration of two modified-release formulations in healthy adults. Clin Pharmacokinet 42:393–401, 2003

Masand PS, Tesar GE: Use of stimulants in the medically ill. Psychiatr Clin North Am 19:515–547, 1996

Masand PS, Anand VS, Tanquary JF: Psychostimulant augmentation of second generation antidepressants: a case series. Depress Anxiety 7:89–91, 1998

McCracken JT, Biederman J, Greenhill LL, et al: Analog classroom assessment of a once-daily mixed amphetamine formulation, SLI381 (Adderall XR), in children with ADHD. J Am Acad Child Adolesc Psychiatry 42:673–683, 2003

McGough JJ, Biederman J, Wigal SB, et al: Long-term tolerability and effectiveness of once-daily mixed amphetamine salts (Adderall XR) in children with ADHD. J Am Acad Child Adolesc Psychiatry 44:530–538, 2005a

McGough JJ, Pataki CS, Suddath R: Dexmethylphenidate extended-release capsules for attention deficit hyperactivity disorder. Expert Rev Neurother 5:437–441, 2005b

Methylin Chewable Tablets (package insert). St. Louis, MO, Mallinckrodt Inc, 2004

Methylin Oral Solution (package insert). St. Louis, MO, Mallinckrodt Inc, 2004

Meyers CA, Weitzner MA, Valentine AD, et al: Methylphenidate therapy improves cognition, mood, and function of brain tumor patients. J Clin Oncol 16:2522–2527, 1998

Michelson D, Faries D, Wernicke J, et al: Atomoxetine in the treatment of children and adolescents with attention-deficit/hyperactivity disorder: a randomized, placebo-controlled, dose-response study. Pediatrics 108:E83; 2001

Michelson D, Allen AJ, Busner J, et al: Once-daily atomoxetine treatment for children and adolescents with attention deficit hyperactivity disorder: a randomized, placebo-controlled study. Am J Psychiatry 159:1896–1901, 2002

Michelson D, Adler L, Spencer T, et al: Atomoxetine in adults with ADHD: two randomized, placebo-controlled studies. Biol Psychiatry 53:112–120, 2003

Michelson D, Buitelaar JK, Danckaerts M, et al: Relapse prevention in pediatric patients with ADHD treated with atomoxetine: a randomized, double-blind, placebo-controlled study. J Am Acad Child Adolesc Psychiatry 43:896–904, 2004

Mitler MM, Hajdukovic R, Erman M, et al: Narcolepsy. J Clin Neurophysiol 7:93–118, 1990

Mitler MM, Harsh J, Hirshkowitz M, et al: Long-term efficacy and safety of modafinil (Provigil) for the treatment of excessive daytime sleepiness associated with narcolepsy. Sleep Med 1:231–243, 2000

Modi NB, Lindemulder B, Gupta SK: Single- and multiple-dose pharmacokinetics of an oral once-a-day osmotic controlled-release OROS (methylphenidate HCL) formulation. J Clin Pharmacol 40:379–388, 2000a

Modi NB, Wang B, Noveck RJ, et al: Dose-proportional and stereospecific pharmacokinetics of methylphenidate delivered using an osmotic, controlled-release oral delivery system. J Clin Pharmacol 40:1141–1149, 2000b

Olin J, Masand P: Psychostimulants for depression in hospitalized cancer patients. Psychosomatics 37:57–62, 1996

Pelham WE, Sturges J, Hoza J, et al: Sustained release and standard methylphenidate effects on cognitive and social behavior in children with ADHD. Pediatrics 80:491–501, 1987

Pelham WE Jr, Greenslade KE, Vodde-Hamilton M, et al: Relative efficacy of long-acting stimulants on children with attention deficit-hyperactivity disorder: a comparison of standard methylphenidate, sustained-release methylphenidate, sustained-release dextroamphetamine, and pemoline. Pediatrics 86:226–237, 1990

Pelham WE, Gnagy EM, Burrows-Maclean L, et al: Once-a-day Concerta methylphenidate versus three-times-daily methylphenidate in laboratory and natural settings. Pediatrics 107:1–15, 2001

Pentikis HS, Simmons RD, Benedict MF, et al: Methylphenidate bioavailability in adults when an extended-release multiparticulate formulation is administered sprinkled on food or as an intact capsule. J Am Acad Child Adolesc Psychiatry 41:443–449, 2002

Physicians' Desk Reference, 59th Edition. Montvale, NJ, Medical Economics, 2005a

Physicians' Desk Reference, 59th Edition (Supplement A), Montvale, NJ, Medical Economics, 2005b

Rapoport JL, Buchsbaum MS, Weingarter H, et al: Dextroamphetamine: cognitive and behavioral effects in normal and hyperactive boys and normal men. Arch Gen Psychiatry 37:933–943, 1980

Ritalin LA (package insert). East Hanover, NJ, Novartis Pharmaceutical Corp, 2004

Russell V, de Villiers A, Sagvolden T, et al: Differences between electrically, Ritalin-, and D-amphetamine-stimulated release of [^{3}H]dopamine from brain slices suggest impaired vesicular storage of dopamine in an animal model of attention-deficit hyperactivity disorder. Behav Brain Res 94:163–171, 1998

Safer DJ, Zito JM, Gardner JE: Pemoline hepatotoxicity and post marketing surveillance. J Am Acad Child Adolesc Psychiatry 40:622–629, 2001

Santosh PJ, Taylor E: Stimulant drugs. Eur Child Adolesc Psychiatry 9 (suppl 1):127–143, 2000

Sauer JM, Long AJ, Ring B, et al: Atomoxetine hydrochloride: clinical drug-drug interaction prediction and outcome. J Pharmacol Exp Ther 308:410–418, 2004

Silber MH: Sleep disorders. Neurol Clin 19:173–186, 2001

Spencer T, Biederman J, Wilens T, et al: Pharmacotherapy of attention-deficit hyperactivity disorder across the life cycle. J Am Acad Child Adolesc Psychiatry 35:409–432, 1996

Spencer T, Biederman J, Wilens T, et al: Effectiveness and tolerability of atomoxetine in adults with attention deficit hyperactivity disorder. Am J Psychiatry 155:693–695, 1998

Spencer T, Biederman J, Heiligenstein J, et al: An open-label, dose-ranging study of atomoxetine in children with attention deficit hyperactivity disorder. J Child Adolesc Psychopharmacol 11:251–265, 2001

Spencer T, Heiligenstein JH, Biederman J, et al: Results from 2 proof-of-concept, placebo-controlled studies of atomoxetine in children with attention-deficit/hyperactivity disorder. J Clin Psychiatry 63:1140–1147, 2002

Spencer T, Greenhill L, on behalf of the Adolescent Study Group: OROS methylphenidate for the treatment of adolescent attention-deficit/hyperactivity disorder. Presented at the annual meeting of the American Academy of Child and Adolescent Psychiatry, Miami, FL, October 14–19, 2003

Stoll AL, Pillay SS, Diamond L, et al: Methylphenidate augmentation of selective serotonin reuptake inhibitors: a case series. J Clin Psychiatry 57:72–76, 1996

Strattera (package insert). Indianapolis, IN, Eli Lilly and Co, 2005

Swanson JM, Volkow ND: Pharmacokinetic and pharmacodynamic properties of stimulants: implications for the design of new treatments for ADHD. Behav Brain Res 130:73–78, 2002

Swanson J, Gupta S, Lam A, et al: Development of a new once-daily formulation of methylphenidate for the treatment of attention-deficit/hyperactivity disorder: proof of concept and proof of product studies. Arch Gen Psychiatry 60:204–211, 2003

Swanson JM, Wigal SB, Wigal T, et al: A comparison of once-daily extended-release methylphenidate formulations in children with attention-deficit/hyperactivity disorder in the laboratory school (the COMACS Study). Pediatrics 113:e206–e216, 2004

Tulloch SJ, Zhang Y, McLean A, et al: SLI381 (Adderall XR), a two-component, extended-release formulation of mixed amphetamine salts: bioavailability of three test formulations and comparison of fasted, fed, and sprinkled administration. Pharmacotherapy 22:1405–1415, 2002

U.S. Modafinil in Narcolepsy Multicenter Study Group: Randomized trial of modafinil for the treatment of pathological somnolence in narcolepsy. Ann Neurol 43:88–97, 1998

U.S. Modafinil in Narcolepsy Multicenter Study Group: Randomized trial of modafinil as a treatment for the excessive daytime somnolence of narcolepsy. Neurology 54:1166–1175, 2000

Wernicke JF, Kratochvil CJ: Safety profile of atomoxetine in the treatment of children and adolescents with ADHD. J Clin Psychiatry 63 (suppl 12):50–55, 2002

Wigal S, Swanson JM, Feifel D, et al: A double-blind, placebo-controlled trial of dexmethylphenidate hydrochloride and d,l-threo-methylphenidate hydrochloride in children with attention-deficit/hyperactivity disorder. J Am Acad Child Adolesc Psychiatry 43:1406–1414, 2004

Wilens TE, Biederman J: The stimulants. Psychiatr Clin North Am 15:191–222, 1992

Wolraich ML, Greenhill LL, Pelham WE, et al: Randomized, controlled trial of OROS methylphenidate once a day in children with attention-deficit/hyperactivity disorder. Pediatrics 108:883–892, 2001

7

COGNITIVE ENHANCERS

In this chapter, we use the term *cognitive enhancers* to refer to two classes of pharmacological agents used in the treatment of Alzheimer's disease: the cholinesterase inhibitors and the *N*-methyl-D-aspartate (NMDA) receptor antagonists.

■ CHOLINESTERASE INHIBITORS

Cholinesterase inhibitors are the current standard of care in the pharmacological management of mild to moderate dementia of the Alzheimer's type. Benefits of these agents include the preservation of functioning, slowing of cognitive decline, and delay in nursing home placement (see reviews by Cummings 2003; Doody et al. 2001b; Ellis 2005; Schneider 2001). The cholinesterase inhibitors currently available in the United States are outlined in Table 7–1.

Mechanisms of Action

Cholinesterase inhibitors cross the blood-brain barrier and decrease enzymatic hydrolysis of acetylcholine in the synaptic cleft, thereby increasing acetylcholine availability for neurotransmission. The rationale for using cholinergic agents to treat Alzheimer's disease stems from evidence of decreased cerebral choline acetyltransferase (the enzyme responsible for acetylcholine synthesis) and cholinergic neuron loss in the nucleus basalis of Meynert, which correlate with plaque formation and cognitive impairment (Arendt et al. 1985; Davies and Maloney 1976; Etienne et al. 1986; Perry et al. 1978b).

TABLE 7–1. Cholinesterase inhibitors available in the United States

Drug	Trade name	Dosing guidelines	Formulations
Tacrine	Cognex	Administer 10 mg po qid for 4 weeks, then 20 mg qid for 4 weeks, then 30 mg qid for 4 weeks, and then 40 mg qid. Titration is based on tolerability and serum transaminase levels. Refer to current product labeling for guidelines on dose adjustments, monitoring, and rechallenging.	10-, 20-, 30-, 40-mg capsules
Donepezil	Aricept	Administer 5 mg po qhs (with or without a meal) for 4–6 weeks. Some patients then increase to 10 mg/day if tolerated. Target daily dose range: 5–10 mg po qhs	5-, 10-mg tablets 5-, 10-mg oral disintegrating tablets (Aricept ODT)
Rivastigmine	Exelon	Administer 1.5 mg po bid (preferably with meals) for 4 weeks, then increase in increments of 1.5 mg/dose every 2–4 weeks, as tolerated, to a maximum dose of 6 mg po bid. Target daily dose range: 3–6 mg po bid	1.5-, 3-, 4.5-, 6-mg capsules 2 mg/mL oral solution (in bottles of 120-mL with dosing syringe)
Galantamine	Razadyne	Administer 4 mg po bid (preferably with meals) for at least 4 weeks, then increase to an initial target dose of 8 mg bid for at least 4 weeks. If tolerated, the dose may then be further increased to 12 mg bid. Target daily dose range: 8–12 mg po bid	4-, 8-, 12-mg tablets 4 mg/mL oral solution (in 100-mL bottle with calibrated pipette)

TABLE 7–1. Cholinesterase inhibitors available in the United States (continued)

Drug	Trade name	Dosing guidelines	Formulations
	Razadyne ER	Administer 8 mg po qam (preferably with meals) for at least 4 weeks, then increase to an initial target dose of 16 mg po qam for at least an additional 4 weeks. If this is tolerated, a further dose increase to 12 mg bid or 24 mg po qam may then be attempted. Target daily dose range: 16–24 mg po qam	8-, 16-, 24-mg capsules

Note.   po=orally; qid=four times daily; qhs=every night before bedtime; bid=twice daily; qam=every morning.
Source.   Aricept 2005; Doody et al. 2001b; Physicians' Desk Reference 2005; Razadyne 2005; Razadyne ER 2005; Schneider 2001.

Individual cholinesterase inhibitors differ in their selectivity, mechanism of inhibition of acetylcholinesterase (Schneider 2001), and pharmacokinetic properties (outlined in Table 7–2).

Clinical Use

Dosing guidelines are shown in Table 7–1. Higher doses tend to be more effective than lower doses (Schneider 2001) but also may be associated with more side effects. Treatment should be considered as early as possible after Alzheimer's disease has been diagnosed. Although numerous differences in pharmacological and pharmacokinetic properties among the available cholinesterase inhibitors exist, the clinical significance of these differences with respect to the treatment of Alzheimer's disease has yet to be determined. Thus, donepezil, galantamine, and rivastigmine each can be considered a reasonable first-choice medication.

Although these agents are currently indicated for the treatment of mild to moderate Alzheimer's disease, there is considerable interest in evaluating these agents in more advanced stages of the disease (Blesa et al. 2003; Bullock et al. 2005; Feldman et al. 2003; Gauthier et al. 2002; Karaman et al. 2005).

Common side effects include nausea, vomiting, abdominal pain, diarrhea, and dizziness. These side effects tend to be associated with treatment initiation or early dose increases and are often transient. Anorexia and weight loss also may occur and may persist throughout treatment. Potentially dangerous side effects include myasthenia, respiratory depression, and bradycardia. Dose reduction or medication discontinuation should be considered if serious side effects occur.

All cholinesterase inhibitors should be used with caution in patients with cardiac conduction problems because vagotonic effects can lead to bradycardia. In addition, caution is warranted in patients with comorbid asthma, chronic obstructive pulmonary disease, bladder outlet obstruction, or seizures, as well as in patients at risk for gastrointestinal ulcers or bleeding (Fuller and Sajatovic 2000).

In general, patients who miss several consecutive doses of cholinesterase inhibitors should resume treatment at the recommended

TABLE 7–2. Pharmacokinetics and key features of cholinesterase inhibitors

Drug	Protein binding	Half-life (hours)	Relations to cytochrome P450 (CYP) system	Other key features
Tacrine	55%	2–4	CYP 1A2 substrate CYP 1A2 inhibitor	Rarely used in current clinical practice Risk for hepatotoxicity Multiple doses daily Requires close hepatic monitoring
Donepezil	>95%	70	CYP 2D6 substrate CYP 3A4 substrate	Once-daily dosing
Rivastigmine	40%	1.5	None anticipated	Not hepatically metabolized (metabolized by hydrolysis and renally eliminated) Dual acetylcholinesterase and butyrylcholinesterase inhibitor
Galantamine	18%	7	CYP 2D6 substrate CYP 3A4 substrate	Allosteric nicotinic receptor activity Once-daily dosing for extended-release formulation

Source. Aricept 2005; Bores et al. 1996; Fuller and Sajatovic 2000; Physicians' Desk Reference 2005; Razadyne 2005; Razadyne ER 2005; Watkins et al. 1994.

starting dose, and the dose should be subsequently titrated according to recommended guidelines.

The optimal duration of treatment with cholinesterase inhibitors has not been definitively established. Most randomized controlled trials in patients with mild to moderate Alzheimer's disease have been 26 weeks in duration or less. However, some data (mostly open-label continuation data of placebo-controlled trials) suggest continued benefits with treatment for 1 year or longer (Bullock and Dengiz 2005; Doody et al. 2001a; Farlow et al. 2000; Grossberg et al. 2004; Lyketsos et al. 2004; Mohs et al. 2001; Pirttila et al. 2004; Raskind et al. 2000, 2004; Rogers et al. 2000; Small et al. 2005; Wilcock et al. 2003; Winblad et al. 2001).

If a patient's symptoms have an inadequate treatment response to one cholinesterase inhibitor, a trial of a different agent within the class may be beneficial (Auriacombe et al. 2002). An expert consensus panel met in 2002 to discuss the clinical importance of switching cholinesterase inhibitors and subsequently published a summary consensus article (Gauthier et al. 2003). In short, they advised that patients should be switched from one cholinesterase to another only if they lack an initial treatment response, experience a loss of efficacy after an initial response, or experience safety or tolerability issues. If dose adjustments are unsuccessful in addressing these issues, then a medication switch should be considered after a minimum treatment period of 6 months with the initial agent (Gauthier et al. 2003). The optimal procedure for switching between agents is unclear. One author recently proposed a washout period of five half-lives from the first medication before introducing the second agent to minimize the potential for adverse interactions (Cummings 2003).

Clinicians often use each cholinesterase inhibitor in combination with memantine; however, the best evidence to date for such combination treatment is the use of memantine in patients with moderate to severe Alzheimer's disease already taking donepezil (Tariot et al. 2004).

Donepezil

Donepezil is a selective, reversible inhibitor of acetylcholinesterase. Its long half-life allows for once-daily dosing. Several studies have confirmed the efficacy of donepezil, compared with placebo, in improving cognition and maintaining global functioning in patients with mild to moderate Alzheimer's disease during acute treatment (Burns et al. 1999; Rogers and Friedhoff 1996; Rogers et al. 1998a, 1998b; Tariot et al. 2001), as well as potential benefits with long-term treatment (Mohs et al. 2001; Rogers et al. 2000; Winblad et al. 2001). A double-blind, placebo-controlled, survival study of donepezil in 415 patients with Alzheimer's disease showed a significant reduction in the risk of functional decline over the 54-week study period (Mohs et al. 2001). In this study, the time to clinically evident functional decline was delayed by a median of 5 months in the donepezil-treated group compared with the placebo group. An 18-month open study in a clinical practice setting showed sustained improvement in cognitive and neuropsychiatric symptoms in some patients with mild to moderate dementia (Matthews et al. 2000). In a 24-week controlled trial of donepezil in 290 participants with moderate to severe Alzheimer's disease, the drug had beneficial effects on cognition and behavior and aided stabilization of functioning (Feldman et al. 2001).

Donepezil is currently approved by the U.S. Food and Drug Administration (FDA) only for the treatment of mild to moderate Alzheimer's disease, but its efficacy also has been examined in other dementias, including moderate to severe Alzheimer's disease (Feldman et al. 2003; Gauthier et al. 2002), Parkinson's disease (Aarsland et al. 2002; Leroi et al. 2004; Ravina et al. 2005), and vascular dementia (Black et al. 2003; Wilkinson et al. 2003). Further study in these areas is needed.

Risks, Side Effects, and Their Management

Common side effects include nausea, vomiting, diarrhea, abdominal pain, anorexia, weight loss, insomnia, and fatigue. Some patients also may experience muscle cramps, dizziness, and syncope.

Drug Interactions

Donepezil is metabolized by cytochrome P450 (CYP) 2D6 and 3A4. Inhibitors of either enzyme can increase donepezil levels, and inducers can decrease donepezil levels. All cholinesterase inhibitors can exaggerate the effects of succinylcholine-like muscle relaxants during anesthesia. Use of cholinesterase inhibitors in combination with other cholinergic agents, such as bethanechol, can lead to synergistic effects and increased toxicity. Concomitant use of anticholinergic agents and cholinesterase inhibitors can decrease the effectiveness of both agents.

Rivastigmine

Rivastigmine is a reversible acetylcholinesterase inhibitor that is relatively selective for an acetylcholinesterase subtype found on postsynaptic membranes. It is also an inhibitor of butyrylcholinesterase, which is largely of glial origin. Both acetylcholinesterase (largely neuronal in origin) and butyrylcholinesterase are active in the breakdown of acetylcholine in normal brains and brains of those with Alzheimer's disease (Mesulam et al. 2002). Additionally, acetylcholinesterase levels progressively decline and butyrylcholinesterase levels increase as Alzheimer's disease progresses (Perry et al. 1978a). Thus, butyrylcholinesterase may be an important target in the treatment of Alzheimer's disease, although studies are needed to determine whether rivastigmine's clinical efficacy differs from that of other cholinesterase inhibitors.

Several placebo-controlled trials have reported rivastigmine's efficacy in improving cognition and functioning in patients with mild to moderate Alzheimer's disease (Corey-Bloom et al. 1998; Forette et al. 1999; Rosler et al. 1999), with recent data suggesting cognitive benefits for up to 2 years (Grossberg et al. 2004). As with donepezil, there has been research interest in examining the efficacy of rivastigmine in other dementia populations, including patients with Parkinson's disease (Emre et al. 2004), advanced moderate Alzheimer's disease (Karaman et al. 2005), vascular dementia (Moretti et al. 2002, 2003), Alzheimer's dementia with concurrent hypertension or vascular risk factors (Erkinjuntti et al. 2002b; Kumar et al. 2000), and Lewy body dementia (McKeith et al. 2000; Wesnes et al. 2002).

Risks, Side Effects, and Their Management

Common side effects include nausea, vomiting, and weight loss, especially with high-dose treatment. Data suggest that side effects may be decreased by titrating no faster than 1.5 mg twice daily every 2 weeks (Vellas et al. 1998). Severe vomiting may occur if rivastigmine therapy is resumed after a treatment interruption. Therefore, patients resuming rivastigmine therapy after several days or more should begin with the recommended starting dose and follow the titration schedule.

Drug Interactions

Because rivastigmine is not hepatically metabolized, pharmacokinetic cytochrome P450–related drug interactions are not expected. However, the previously discussed pharmacodynamic interactions associated with other cholinesterase inhibitors may occur with rivastigmine as well.

Galantamine

Galantamine is a competitive, reversible cholinesterase inhibitor and an allosteric modulator of presynaptic nicotinic receptors, thereby enhancing synaptic acetylcholine activity (Bores et al. 1996; Scott and Goa 2000). Double-blind, placebo-controlled studies have reported galantamine's efficacy in improving cognition and functional impairment in patients with mild to moderate Alzheimer's disease (Raskind et al. 2000; Rockwood et al. 2001; Suh et al. 2004; Tariot et al. 2000; Wilcock et al. 2000). Recent data suggest that continued galantamine treatment may be associated with sustained cognitive benefits for up to 36 months (Lyketsos et al. 2004; Pirttila et al. 2004; Raskind et al. 2004).

Galantamine HBr was marketed under the brand name Reminyl. The name was changed in 2005 to Razadyne to avoid confusion with the diabetes drug Amaryl (glimeperide).

Galantamine, like other cholinesterase inhibitors, is currently approved by the FDA only for the treatment of mild to moderate

Alzheimer's disease; however, studies have investigated its potential utility in vascular dementia (Erkinjuntti et al. 2002a) and advanced moderate Alzheimer's disease (Blesa et al. 2003).

Risks, Side Effects, and Their Management

Common side effects reported in clinical trials include nausea, vomiting, diarrhea, anorexia, weight loss, dizziness, abdominal pain, and tremor. Most side effects tend to be dose related and may be decreased with a slow titration schedule of 4 mg twice daily every 4 weeks. Dosing should be done cautiously in patients with moderate renal or hepatic impairment, and galantamine should be avoided in those with severe impairment.

Drug Interactions

Galantamine is metabolized primarily by CYP 2D6 and 3A4, and levels may be altered by inducers or inhibitors of these enzymes. Galantamine has not been shown to inhibit major cytochrome P450 enzymes. However, the pharmacodynamic interactions associated with other cholinesterase inhibitors may occur.

Tacrine

Tacrine was the first cholinesterase inhibitor to be approved by the FDA for the treatment of mild to moderate dementia. Numerous studies have shown its efficacy in mild to moderate Alzheimer's disease (Chatellier and Lacomblez 1990; Davis et al. 1992; Eagger et al. 1991; Farlow et al. 1992; Gauthier et al. 1990; Knapp et al. 1994). However, because of the risk of hepatotoxicity (Watkins et al. 1994), tacrine use has become exceedingly rare, and tacrine is not considered a first-line agent. Serum transaminase levels must be monitored every 2 weeks from at least week 4 to week 16 after initiation of tacrine treatment. In controlled trials of tacrine for the treatment of dementia, up to 50% of the patients taking high-dose tacrine had increased transaminase levels (see review by Doody et al. 2001b), and 25% had increases in alanine aminotransferase concentrations beyond three times the upper limit of normal (Grundman and Thal

2000). Increases in alanine aminotransferase levels require dose decreases and more frequent monitoring of hepatic function.

■ NMDA RECEPTOR ANTAGONISTS

Memantine

Memantine is currently the only medication approved by the FDA for the treatment of moderate to severe dementia of the Alzheimer's type (Reisberg et al. 2003; Winblad and Poritis 1999). Although its use also has been investigated in patients with mild to moderate vascular dementia (Orgogozo et al. 2002; Wilcock et al. 2002), this specific use has not yet been approved.

Mechanism of Action

Persistent excitatory glutamatergic stimulation of postsynaptic NMDA receptors, which may cause neuronal toxicity by allowing excessive calcium entry into neurons, has been implicated in the symptomatology of dementia of the Alzheimer's type (Farber et al. 1998). Memantine is a moderate-affinity, noncompetitive inhibitor of NMDA receptors (Danysz et al. 2000).

Clinical Use

Memantine was approved by the FDA in October 2003 for the treatment of moderate to severe dementia of the Alzheimer's type. Its efficacy has been shown in placebo-controlled trials when taken as a monotherapy (Reisberg et al. 2003; Winblad and Poritis 1999) or in patients receiving stable donepezil therapy (Tariot et al. 2004). It is currently available in 5- and 10-mg tablets, and doses can be administered with or without meals.

The typical starting dose is 5 mg/day. Subsequent dose increases should occur in 5-mg increments (at least 1 week apart) to a target dose of 10 mg twice daily (or 5 mg twice daily in patients with renal impairment). Doses greater than the initial 5-mg starting dose should be divided into two daily doses (Namenda 2005).

Pharmacokinetics

Memantine is well absorbed after oral administration, is not highly protein bound, and has a half-life of 60–80 hours. Memantine is primarily renally excreted unchanged in the urine; however, a portion of the administered dose is converted to three inactive metabolites. The cytochrome P450 system does not play a key role in its metabolism (Namenda 2005).

Risks, Side Effects, and Their Management

Memantine was generally well tolerated in clinical trials assessing its use in Alzheimer's disease, with no major differences in tolerability from placebo (Reisberg et al. 2003; Winblad and Poritis 1999). The side effects most commonly reported with memantine use in placebo-controlled trials include dizziness, headache, confusion, constipation, coughing, hypertension, somnolence, pain, vomiting, and hallucinations. No significant changes were noted in vital signs, serum chemistry of hematology laboratory studies, or electrocardiogram parameters (Namenda 2005). Because memantine is partly excreted unchanged by the kidneys, clinicians are advised to use lower doses in patients with renal impairment and to avoid use in patients with severe renal impairment.

Drug Interactions

Memantine is not a major substrate for hepatic cytochrome P450 isoenzymes and has not been shown to significantly inhibit or induce these enzymes. However, memantine is partially excreted by renal tubular secretion. Thus, concomitant use of other medications that use the same renal system (i.e., triampterene, hydrochlorothiazide, digoxin, cimetidine, ranitidine, metformin, and quinidine) may affect plasma levels of both drugs (Namenda 2005). Memantine should not be used in combination with other NMDA receptor antagonists, such as amantadine or dextromethorphan, because these combinations have not been formally studied. The clearance of memantine can be reduced when the urine is alkalinized, such as with the concomitant use of sodium bicarbonate or carbonic anhydrase inhibitors or during severe urinary tract infections (Namenda 2005).

■ REFERENCES

Aarsland D, Laake K, Larsen JP, et al: Donepezil for cognitive impairment in Parkinson's disease: a randomized, controlled study. J Neurol Neurosurg Psychiatry 72:708–712, 2002

Arendt T, Bigl V, Tennstedt A, et al: Neuronal loss in different parts of the nucleus basalis is related to neuritic plaque formation in cortical target areas in Alzheimer's disease. Neuroscience 14:1–14, 1985

Aricept (prescribing information). Teaneck, NJ, Eisai Co Ltd, 2005

Auriacombe S, Pere JJ, Loria-Kanza Y, et al: Efficacy and safety of rivastigmine in patients with Alzheimer's disease who failed to benefit from treatment with donepezil. Curr Med Res Opin 18:129–138, 2002

Black S, Roman GC, Geldmacher DS, et al: Efficacy and tolerability of donepezil in vascular dementia: positive results of a 24-week, multicenter, international, randomized, placebo-controlled clinical trial. Stroke 34:2323–2330, 2003

Blesa R, Davidson M, Kurz A, et al: Galantamine provides sustained benefits in patients with 'advanced moderate' Alzheimer's disease for at least 12 months. Dement Geriatr Cogn Disord 15:79–87, 2003

Bores GM, Huger FP, Petko W, et al: Pharmacological evaluation of novel Alzheimer's disease therapeutics: acetylcholinesterase inhibitors related to galanthamine. J Pharmacol Exp Ther 277:728–738, 1996

Bullock R, Dengiz A: Cognitive performance in patients with Alzheimer's disease receiving cholinesterase inhibitors for up to 5 years. Int J Clin Pract 59:817–822, 2005

Bullock R, Touchon J, Bergman H, et al: Rivastigmine and donepezil treatment in moderate to moderately severe Alzheimer's disease over a 2 year period. Curr Med Res Opin 21:1317–1327, 2005

Burns A, Rossor M, Hecker J, et al: The effects of donepezil in Alzheimer's disease—results from a multinational trial. Dement Geriatr Cogn Disord 10:237–244, 1999

Chatellier G, Lacomblez L: Tacrine (tetrahydroaminoacridine; THA) and lecithin in senile dementia of the Alzheimer's type: a multicentre trial. Groupe Français d'Étude de la Tétrahydroaminoacridine. BMJ 300:495–499, 1990

Corey-Bloom J, Anand R, Veach J, et al: A randomized trial evaluating the efficacy and safety of ENA 713 (rivastigmine tartrate), a new acetylcholinesterase inhibitor, in patients with mild to moderate Alzheimer's disease. The ENA 713 B352 Study Group. Int J Geriatr Psychopharmacol 1:55–65, 1998

Cummings JL: Use of cholinesterase inhibitors in clinical practice: evidence-based recommendations. Am J Geriatr Psychiatry 11:131–145, 2003

Danysz W, Parsons CG, Mobius HJ, et al: Neuroprotective and symptomalogical action of memantine relevant for Alzheimer's disease—a unified glutamatergic hypothesis on the mechanism of action. Neurotox Res 2:85–98, 2000

Davies P, Maloney AJ: Selective loss of central cholinergic neurons in Alzheimer's disease (letter). Lancet 2:1403, 1976

Davis KL, Thal LJ, Gamzu ER, et al: A double-blind, placebo-controlled multicenter study of tacrine for Alzheimer's disease. The Tacrine Collaborative Study Group. N Engl J Med 327:1253–1259, 1992

Doody RS, Geldmacher DS, Gordon B, et al: Open-label, multi-center, phase 3 extension study of the safety and efficacy of donepezil in patients with Alzheimer disease. Arch Neurol 58:427–433, 2001a

Doody RS, Stevens JC, Beck C, et al: Practice parameter: management of dementia (an evidence-based review). Report of the Quality Standards Subcommittee of the American Academy of Neurology. Neurology 56:1154–1166, 2001b

Eagger SA, Levy R, Sahakian BJ: Tacrine in Alzheimer's disease. Lancet 337:989–992, 1991

Ellis JM: Cholinesterase inhibitors in the treatment of dementia. J Am Osteopath Assoc 105:145–158, 2005

Emre M, Aarsland D, Albanese A, et al: Rivastigmine for dementia associated with Parkinson's disease. N Engl J Med 351:2509–2518, 2004

Erkinjuntti T, Kurz A, Gauthier S, et al: Efficacy of galantamine in probable vascular dementia and Alzheimer's disease combined with cerebrovascular disease: a randomized trial. Lancet 359:1283–1290, 2002a

Erkinjuntti T, Skoog I, Lane R, et al: Rivastigmine in patients with Alzheimer's disease and concurrent hypertension. Int J Clin Pract 56:791–796, 2002b

Etienne P, Robitaille Y, Wood P, et al: Nucleus basalis neuronal loss, neuritic plaques and choline acetyltransferase activity in advanced Alzheimer's disease. Neuroscience 19:1279–1291, 1986

Farber NB, Newcomer JW, Olney JW: The glutamate synapse in neuropsychiatric disorders: focus on schizophrenia and Alzheimer's disease. Prog Brain Res 116:421–437, 1998

Farlow M, Gracon SI, Hershey LA, et al: A controlled trial of tacrine in Alzheimer's disease. The Tacrine Study Group. JAMA 268:2523–2529, 1992

Farlow M, Anand R, Messina J Jr, et al: A 52-week study of the efficacy of rivastigmine in patients with mild to moderately severe Alzheimer's disease. Eur Neurol 44:231–241, 2000

Feldman H, Gauthier S, Hecker J, et al: A 24-week, randomized, double-blind study of donepezil in moderate to severe Alzheimer's disease. The Donepezil MSAD Study Investigators Group. Neurology 57:613–620, 2001

Feldman H, Gauthier S, Hecker J, et al: Efficacy of donepezil on maintenance of activities of daily living with moderate to severe Alzheimer's disease and the effect on caregiver burden. J Am Geriatr Soc 51:737–744, 2003

Forette F, Anand R, Gharabawi G: A phase II study in patients with Alzheimer's disease to assess the preliminary efficacy and maximum tolerated dose of rivastigmine (Exelon). Eur J Neurol 6:423–429, 1999

Fuller MA, Sajatovic M: Psychotropic Drug Information Handbook. Hudson, OH, Lexi-Comp, 2000

Gauthier S, Bouchard R, Lamontagne A, et al: Tetrahydroaminoacridine-lecithin combination treatment in patients with intermediate-stage Alzheimer's disease: results of a Canadian double-blind, crossover, multicenter study. N Engl J Med 322:1272–1276, 1990

Gauthier S, Feldman H, Hecker J, et al: Efficacy of donepezil on behavioral symptoms in patients with moderate to severe Alzheimer's disease. Int Psychogeriatr 14:389–401, 2002

Gauthier S, Emre M, Farlow MR, et al: Strategies for continued successful treatment of Alzheimer's disease: switching cholinesterase inhibitors. Curr Med Res Opin 19:707–714, 2003

Grossberg G, Irwin P, Satlin A, et al: Rivastigmine in Alzheimer's disease: efficacy over two years. Am J Geriatr Psychiatry 12:420–431, 2004

Grundman M, Thal LJ: Treatment of Alzheimer's disease: rationale and strategies. Neurol Clin 18:807–828, 2000

Karaman Y, Erdogan F, Koseoglu E, et al: A 12-month study of the efficacy of rivastigmine in patients with advanced moderate Alzheimer's disease. Dement Geriatr Cogn Disord 19:51–56, 2005

Knapp MJ, Knopman DS, Solomon PR, et al: A 30-week randomized controlled trial of high-dose tacrine in patients with Alzheimer's disease. The Tacrine Study Group. JAMA 271:985–991, 1994

Kumar V, Anand R, Messina J, et al: An efficacy and safety analysis of Exelon in Alzheimer's disease with concurrent vascular risk factors. Eur J Neurol 7:159–169, 2000

Leroi I, Brandt J, Reich SG, et al: Randomized, placebo-controlled trial of donepezil in cognitive impairment in Parkinson's disease. Int J Geriatr Psychiatry 19:1–8, 2004

Lyketsos CG, Reichman WE, Kershaw P, et al: Long-term outcomes of galantamine treatment in patients with Alzheimer disease. Am J Geriatr Psychiatry 12:473–482, 2004

Matthews HP, Korbey J, Wilkinson DG, et al: Donepezil in Alzheimer's disease: eighteen month results from Southampton Memory Clinic. Int J Geriatr Psychiatry 15:713–720, 2000

McKeith I, Del Ser T, Spano P, et al: Efficacy of rivastigmine in dementia with Lewy bodies: a randomized, double-blind, placebo-controlled international study. Lancet 356:2031–2036, 2000

Mesulam M, Guillozet A, Shaw P, et al: Widely spread butyrylcholinesterase can hydrolyze acetylcholine in the normal and Alzheimer brain. Neurobiol Dis 9:88–93, 2002

Mohs RC, Doody RS, Morris JC, et al: A 1-year, placebo-controlled preservation of function survival study of donepezil in AD patients. Neurology 57:481–488, 2001

Moretti R, Torre P, Antonello RM, et al: Rivastigmine in subcortical vascular dementia: an open 22-month study. J Neurol Sci 203:141–146, 2002

Moretti R, Torre P, Antonello RM, et al: Rivastigmine in subcortical vascular dementia: a randomized, controlled, open 12-month study in 208 patients. Am J Alzheimers Dis Other Demen 18:265–272, 2003

Namenda (prescribing information). St. Louis, MO, Forest Pharmaceuticals Inc, 2005

Orgogozo J-M, Rigaud A-S, Stoffler A, et al: Efficacy and safety of memantine in patients with mild to moderate vascular dementia: a randomized, placebo-controlled trial (MMM300). Stroke 3:1834–1839, 2002

Perry EK, Perry RH, Blessed G, et al: Changes in brain cholinesterases in senile dementia of Alzheimer type. Neuropathol Appl Neurobiol 4:273–277, 1978a

Perry EK, Tomlinson BE, Blessed G, et al: Correlation of cholinergic abnormalities with senile plaques and mental test scores in senile dementia. BMJ 2:1457–1459, 1978b

Physicians' Desk Reference, 59th Edition. Montvale, NJ, Medical Economics, 2005

Pirttila T, Wilcock G, Truyen L, et al: Long-term efficacy and safety of galantamine in patients with mild-to-moderate Alzheimer's disease: multicenter trial. Eur J Neurol 11:734–741, 2004

Raskind MA, Peskind ER, Wessel T, et al: Galantamine in AD: a 6-month randomized, placebo-controlled trial with a 6-month extension. The Galantamine USA-1 Study Group. Neurology 54:2261–2268, 2000

Raskind MA, Peskind ER, Truyen L, et al: The cognitive benefits of galantamine are sustained for at least 36 months: a long-term extension trial. Arch Neurol 61:252–256, 2004

Ravina B, Putt M, Siderowf A, et al: Donepezil for dementia in Parkinson's disease: a randomised, double blind, placebo controlled, crossover study. J Neurol Neurosurg Psychiatry 76:934–939, 2005

Razadyne (prescribing information). Titusville, NJ, Ortho-McNeil Neurologics Inc, 2005

Razadyne ER (prescribing information). Titusville, NJ, Ortho-McNeil Neurologics Inc, 2005

Reisberg B, Doody R, Stoffler A, et al: Memantine in moderate-to-severe Alzheimer's disease. N Engl J Med 348:1333–1341, 2003

Rockwood K, Mintzer J, Truyen L, et al: Effects of a flexible galantamine dose in Alzheimer's disease: a randomized, controlled trial. J Neurol Neurosurg Psychiatry 71:589–595, 2001

Rogers SL, Friedhoff LT: The efficacy and safety of donepezil in patients with Alzheimer's disease: results of a U.S. multicentre, randomized, double-blind, placebo-controlled trial. The Donepezil Study Group. Dementia 7:293–303, 1996

Rogers SL, Doody RS, Mohs RC, et al: Donepezil improves cognition and global function in Alzheimer's disease: a 15-week, double-blind, placebo-controlled study. The Donepezil Study Group. Arch Intern Med 158:1021–1031, 1998a

Rogers SL, Farlow MR, Doody RS, et al: A 24-week, double-blind, placebo-controlled trial of donepezil in patients with Alzheimer's disease. The Donepezil Study Group. Neurology 50:136–145, 1998b

Rogers SL, Doody RS, Pratt RD, et al: Long-term efficacy and safety of donepezil in the treatment of Alzheimer's disease: final analysis of a US multicentre open-label study. Eur Neuropsychopharmacol 10:195–203, 2000

Rosler M, Anand R, Cicin-Sain A, et al: Efficacy and safety of rivastigmine in patients with Alzheimer's disease: international randomised controlled trial. BMJ 318:633–638, 1999

Schneider LS: Treatment of Alzheimer's disease with cholinesterase inhibitors. Clin Geriatr Med 17:337–358, 2001

Scott LJ, Goa KL: Galantamine: a review of its use in Alzheimer's disease. Drugs 60:1095–1122, 2000

Small G, Kaufer K, Mendiondo MS, et al: Cognitive performance in Alzheimer's disease patients receiving rivastigmine for up to 5 years. Int J Clin Pract 59:473–477, 2005

Suh GH, Yeon Jung H, Uk Lee C, et al: A prospective, double-blind, community-controlled comparison of three doses of galantamine in the treatment of mild to moderate Alzheimer's disease in a Korean population. Clin Ther 26:1608–1618, 2004

Tariot PN, Solomon PR, Morris JC, et al: A 5-month, randomized, placebo-controlled trial of galantamine in AD. The Galantamine USA-10 Study Group. Neurology 54:2269–2276, 2000

Tariot PN, Cummings JL, Katz IR, et al: A randomized, double-blind, placebo-controlled study of the efficacy and safety of donepezil in patients with Alzheimer's disease in the nursing home setting. J Am Geriatr Soc 49:1590–1599, 2001

Tariot PN, Farlow MR, Grossberg GT, et al: Memantine treatment in patients with moderate to severe Alzheimer disease already receiving donepezil: a randomized controlled trial. JAMA 291:317–324, 2004

Vellas B, Inglis F, Potkin S: Interim results from an international clinical trial with rivastigmine evaluating a 2-week titration rate in mild to severe Alzheimer's patients. Int J Geriatr Psychopharmacol 1:140–144, 1998

Watkins PB, Zimmerman HJ, Knapp MJ, et al: Hepatotoxic effects of tacrine administration in patients with Alzheimer's disease. JAMA 271:992–998, 1994

Wesnes KA, McKeith IG, Ferrara R, et al: Effects of rivastigmine on cognitive function in dementia with Lewy bodies: a randomized placebo-controlled international study using the cognitive research computerized assessment system. Dement Geriatr Cogn Disord 13:183–192, 2002

Wilcock GK, Lilienfeld S, Gaens E: Efficacy and safety of galantamine in patients with mild to moderate Alzheimer's disease: multicentre randomised controlled trial. Galantamine International-1 Study Group. BMJ 321:1445–1449, 2000

Wilcock G, Mobius HJ, Stoffler A, et al: A double-blind, placebo-controlled multicentre study of memantine in mild to moderate vascular dementia (MMM500). Int Clin Psychopharmacol 17:297–305, 2002

Wilcock G, Howe I, Coles H, et al: A long-term comparison of galantamine and donepezil in the treatment of Alzheimer's disease. Drug Aging 20:777–789, 2003

Wilkinson D, Doody R, Helme R, et al: Donepezil in vascular dementia: a randomized, placebo-controlled study. Neurology 61:479–486, 2003

Winblad B, Poritis N: Memantine in severe dementia: results of the M-BEST study (benefit and efficacy in severely demented patients during treatment with memantine). Int J Geriatr Psychiatry 14:135–146, 1999

Winblad B, Engedal K, Soininen H, et al: A 1 year, randomized, placebo-controlled study of donepezil in patients with mild to moderate AD. Neurology 57:489–495, 2001

Appendix

TRADE/BRAND NAMES OF COMMON PSYCHIATRIC DRUGS

Drug	Trade/brand name
acamprosate calcium	Campral
alprazolam	Xanax, Xanax XR, Niravam
amantadine	Symmetrel
amitriptyline	Elavil
amitriptyline/perphenazine	Triavil
amoxapine	Asendin
amphetamine/dextroamphetamine	Adderall, Adderall XR
aripiprazole	Abilify
atomoxetine	Strattera
benztropine	Cogentin
bromocriptine	Parlodel
bupropion	Wellbutrin, Wellbutrin XL, Wellbutrin SR, Zyban
buspirone	BuSpar
carbamazepine	Tegretol, Epitol, Carbatrol, Equetro
chlordiazepoxide	Librium, Libritabs
chlorpromazine	Thorazine
citalopram	Celexa
clomipramine	Anafranil
clonazepam	Klonopin
clonidine	Catapres
clorazepate	Tranxene
clozapine	Clozaril, FazaClo
dantrolene	Dantrium
desipramine	Norpramin
dexmethylphenidate	Focalin, Focalin XR
dextroamphetamine	Dexedrine, DextroStat
diazepam	Valium
diphenhydramine	Benadryl
divalproex	Depakote, Depakote ER
donepezil	Aricept
doxepin	Sinequan
droperidol	Inapsine
duloxetine	Cymbalta
escitalopram	Lexapro
estazolam	ProSom
eszopiclone	Lunesta

Drug	Trade/brand name
flumazenil	Romazicon
fluoxetine	Prozac, Prozac Weekly, Sarafem
fluphenazine	Prolixin
flurazepam	Dalmane
fluvoxamine	Luvox
gabapentin	Neurontin
galantamine	Razadyne, Razadyne ER
haloperidol	Haldol
hydroxyzine	Atarax, Vistaril
imipramine	Tofranil
isocarboxazid	Marplan
lamotrigine	Lamictal
levetiracetam	Keppra
levothyroxine	Synthroid, Levoxyl, Levothroid
liothyronine	Cytomel
lithium	Eskalith, Eskalith CR, Lithobid
lorazepam	Ativan
loxapine	Loxitane
maprotiline	Ludiomil
memantine	Namenda
meperidine	Demerol
mesoridazine	Serentil
methylphenidate	Ritalin, Ritalin SR, Ritalin LA, Methylin, Methylin ER, Metadate ER, Metadate CD, Concerta
mexiletine	Mexitil
midazolam	Versed
mirtazapine	Remeron
moclobemide	Aurorix, Manerix
modafinil	Provigil
molindone	Moban
naloxone	Narcan
naltrexone	ReVia
nefazodone	Serzone
nifedipine	Adalat
nortriptyline	Pamelor, Aventyl
olanzapine	Zyprexa
olanzapine-fluoxetine	Symbyax

Drug	Trade/brand name
oxazepam	Serax
oxcarbazepine	Trileptal
paroxetine	Paxil, Paxil CR
perphenazine	Trilafon, Etrafon
phenelzine	Nardil
phenobarbital	Luminal
phentolamine	Regitine
phenytoin	Dilantin
physostigmine	Antilirium
pimozide	Orap
pindolol	Visken
pramipexole	Mirapex
propranolol	Inderal
protriptyline	Vivactil
quazepam	Doral
quetiapine	Seroquel
ramelteon	Rozerem
riluzole	Rilutek
risperidone	Risperdal
rivastigmine	Exelon
ropinirole	Requip
selegiline, L-deprenyl	Eldepryl
sertraline	Zoloft
sildenafil	Viagra
tacrine	Cognex
temazepam	Restoril
thioridazine	Mellaril
thiothixene	Navane
thyroxine (levothyroxine)	Synthroid
topiramate	Topamax
tranylcypromine	Parnate
trazodone	Desyrel
triazolam	Halcion
trifluoperazine	Stelazine
trihexyphenidyl	Artane
triiodothyronine (liothyronine)	Cytomel
trimipramine	Surmontil
valproate	*See* valproic acid; divalproex

Drug	Trade/brand name
valproic acid	Depakene
venlafaxine	Effexor, Effexor XR
verapamil	Calan, Isoptin
warfarin	Coumadin
zaleplon	Sonata
ziprasidone	Geodon
zolpidem	Ambien
zonisamide	Zonegran

INDEX

*Page numbers printed in **boldface** type refer to tables or figures.*